Racing Heart

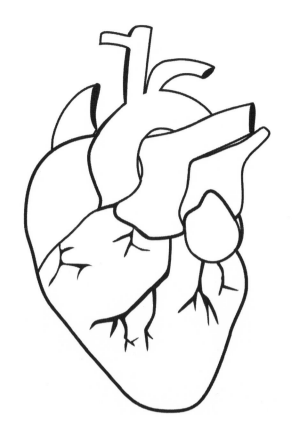

Racing Heart

A RUNNER'S JOURNEY OF LOVE, LOSS AND PERSEVERANCE

Printed in the United States of America

First Printing, 2018

ISBN 978-0-9997950-0-2

Editing by Carol Chesney Hess
Cover design & interior formatting by Noah Adam Paperman

Dedication

I dedicate this book to Dr. Zoubin Alikhani, Dr. Jonathan Kim, and Dr. Shawn Haywood for saving my life in more ways than one. To the community of friends and family who have supported my family and myself every step of the way.

To Brian and Andy for giving me the strength to keep moving forward even when I wasn't sure I wanted to or could. I love you both more than you know.

And lastly, to all those who have lost a piece of themselves because of injury, illness, or for any other reason. I hope this book helps you to find some strength, hope, and grace to move forward no matter what. We are all in this together.

Table of Contents

Acknowledgments

This book would not have been possible without the support and encouragement of my husband, Brian Edwards. His unwavering love and support has allowed me to pursue my passion of helping others in my ways, including writing this book. Without his partnership I would be lost.

Thank you to all of my patients, colleagues, friends, and anyone who listened to me day in and day out as I poured my heart and soul into this book.

Finally, I can't thank my editor, Carol Hess, enough for her guidance, encouragement, enthusiasm, and professional advice along the way. She helped me to believe in myself and my writing.

Introduction

"Everything we are is learned. We learn from experience, from family, friends, and the world around us."

- Unknown

I yell to my husband and son, "I love you," as I rush out of the house, green smoothie and yoga mat in hand. Some mornings it's hard to leave them when they're snuggling up on the couch reading and Andy's giggling. It's a cold Saturday morning in Georgia, and I have my seat warmer on in the car to keep me from shivering. It's around eight, and I'm driving to one of my favorite yoga classes. As I look out the window, I see a runner at the stoplight, dressed in a Boston Marathon jacket. It's so cold, I can see her breath while she runs in place, waiting for the light to change. I think to myself, "She doesn't know how lucky she is. I remember when that used to be me."

My closet is full of running jackets, running hats, running gloves, and running shoes. I have shelves and drawers of race shirts just sitting there, waiting for me to clean them out, but I haven't been able to do it yet. I'm not ready for a life without running gear. I'm not ready for a life without running.

I never imagined there would be a day I wouldn't be able to wake up, throw on my running shoes, and head out the door. The idea of never being able to run again never crossed my mind for even a second. I thought I was going to be that little old lady that shuffled across the finish line on her ninetieth birthday. I know now that won't be me, but knowing it and accepting it aren't the same thing. Not at all.

The light changes. As I drive forward, I look in my rearview mirror and watch the runner cross the street and turn the corner. I wonder where she's going. Is she going to run by my favorite house with the big wraparound porch? Will she run up that steep, really tough hill at the end of the street, or will she decide halfway up she'd rather walk it? How far is she going to run today? Is she meeting her friends for coffee after?

I ran every Saturday morning for years. Some Saturdays, I would get up and meet my girlfriend for a run, and we'd talk about our week. We'd laugh or complain about everything under the sun. Our conversations while running were our therapy, our religion. Other times, my husband and I would go out the door loaded down with the dog, the leash, our son, and the running stroller. And the four of us would spend an hour or two running all over town, enjoying the outdoors and reveling in the time spent together. When we got home, my dog would happily flop down on the floor and pass out for the rest of the day while we made blueberry pancakes. We always made blueberry pancakes. I used to so look forward to those mornings. I still miss them.

A car horn impatiently beeping behind me interrupts my thoughts. This happens a lot these days. I find myself daydreaming about what it feels like to run and what I would be doing if I could still do everything I used to do.

I pull into the parking lot of the yoga studio. I'm the first one here again. I like to arrive early enough to put my mat down in my familiar spot in the room and settle in. I love to feel the sunlight streaming from the skylight above. I enjoy the few moments of peaceful silence before class starts. This morning, as I roll out my mat, I'm not so peaceful. It's because that runner is on my mind.

I still love running. I still love endurance exercise. It was a part of my life for a long time. And now it isn't — or at least not in the same way. I know all too well what it's like to lose what you love. I was forced to change my entire lifestyle in a single moment. Since losing my ability to run and train, I've had to make a lot of lifestyle changes.

I've been forced to look deeper into what is important to me and what I want to get out of this life. It's kind of ironic, but it wasn't until I lost something I loved and depended on that I realized there was another, better version of life I could be living. And slowly my grief at losing one of the great loves of my life is healing.

I discovered that writing was an important part of the healing process for me. I never intended to write a book. But one day I sat down, and I couldn't stop writing. When I finally got up hours later, I felt better. Writing has helped me peel back the layers of what I'm thinking and feeling and see them for what they really are — just thoughts, just feelings. Writing has allowed me to step back and analyze how I *want* to live my life instead of how I *should* live my life. There are more than a million miles between want and should.

Even though I'm only at the beginning of this journey, I should have already died six times. I've survived for a reason. That reason is to share my story of how my life was turned upside down and inside out in a single moment. It's about how I've chosen to move forward even when there were so many times I wasn't sure I could.

I used to be an athlete. In my mind I still am, but my body has decided otherwise. I still crave the run and the endorphins that endurance exercise releases. I miss lots of pieces of my former life and the future life I thought I was going to have, and I'm trying to pick up some of those pieces. But I'm also gathering new pieces and slowly learning to live this new life that I have both been forced to accept and willingly chosen.

In my former life, I was happy, and I thought I had everything I wanted. My husband was my best friend, loving and supportive. I had a beautiful son, and I loved my job and my profession. Then, my life changed dramatically because of circumstances over which I had no control.

We don't always get to choose the turns our lives take. I've learned that, for better or worse, eventually we all go through something that forces us to change the path we are on. Change is never easy, but when it comes, it's our choice how difficult we make it. I could have given up, fought, and denied everything that was going on. Somehow I didn't. Somehow I kept moving forward. Maybe it was instinct as an athlete to finish the race no matter what.

Change is not only difficult, but it's also quite uncomfortable. In fact, some of the most important changes come out of the greatest amount of discomfort. My journey has been full of discomfort and change — the two things I've always hated most. But, when I step back and look at my experience from another perspective, I am surprised to discover that it may have been just exactly what I needed.

My story is deeply entwined with running, but you don't have to be a runner to appreciate my journey. Running isn't just a sport. It's a lifestyle and a community. So losing it has forced me to redefine who I am, how I live, and where I belong. Doesn't everyone have to reexamine themselves and their lives at some point? I think they do.

I never imagined a day when I wouldn't be able to run. To say I love running is a gross understatement. I love the feeling of each foot as it hits the ground, the breeze in my hair, the sweat on my forehead, the peace I experience. I love the way running makes me feel mentally and physically and how it gives me confidence, freedom, and hope. Even every step in my career has been about incorporating the sport I love — from the moment I started running right up until the moment I was told I had to stop.

I ran for more than fourteen years, and it's been more than a year now since I took my last run. I can still close my eyes and imagine myself running my typical five-mile loop in my neighborhood. I can still see the houses that line the route and hear the familiar sounds of kids laughing, dogs barking, and wind rustling in the trees. I can still smell summer's cut grass and autumn's crisp air. I can still remember how each hill felt to climb. I can still see the people I would notice each time I went out.

Giving up my running lifestyle is the hardest thing I've ever done or ever hope to do. I will always miss it. Always.

1

The Running Life

"Running away will never make you free."

- Kenny Loggins

I was raised in upstate New York and Vermont. I don't remember a lot from my childhood, but I do remember a few things from when my parents were still married. I remember things like sitting in the kitchen at a little table while my mom was cooking and baking, like climbing into my brother Luke's hospital bed with him when he was going through cancer treatment to watch *Curious George*, like going with my dad to feed the ducks by the lake in Cooperstown on our way home from the hospital. My parents were cyclists and runners, and I remember their road bikes leaning against the kitchen table and watching them run the Boilermaker 15K Road Race nearly every year.

My parents were both physically active when my brother

and I were really young, but then Luke got sick, and a lot changed. For a few years, we spent most of our weekends at the hospital. My mother often stayed with my brother, and my father took care of me. I didn't really understand what was going on because I was too young. Now that I'm a parent, I understand how a sick child can change you and put a lot of strain on a marriage. My parents got married when they were very young and were only in their early twenties when Luke was diagnosed with cancer. I can't imagine what it would be like to be that young and have to go through such a traumatic event. When my brother finished his treatment and went into remission, my mom and dad split up. I was seven or eight years old, and Luke was five or six.

My mother moved my brother and me to Vermont to start over. She once told me she couldn't stay in New York because she was reminded of when my brother was sick everywhere she went and every time she turned around. I had no idea we were actually moving. While I watched my parents pack up the car, I thought we were going on vacation. Then, as my mother, brother, and I drove away, I looked out the back window of the car. I saw my father sit down on the sidewalk, drop his head into his hands, and begin to cry. I didn't understand why he was so upset or what this meant for us as a family.

When I did finally understand what was going on and realized we weren't ever going back home to New York, I was angry. And I stayed angry for years. I coped by running. Running became a way for me to suppress anger and push through my life without facing all my uncomfortable emotions and experiences.

I understand now that my mom tried her best, but the truth is she was never herself after my brother got sick. There were many nights I could hear her crying. She drank a lot, and she cried a lot. And when she drank, she always cried about my brother being sick and almost dying.

But there were times when things were good. When we cleaned the house, we would turn the music on loud and dance around and have fun. I still remember singing at the top of my lungs and pretending the broom was a guitar. My mom often baked cookies, and she would let us eat the batter. She would make our lunches for school and leave us love notes in our lunch bags or use cookie cutters to turn our sandwiches into stars or hearts. I have some good memories.

However, I have far too many other memories that I spent a lot of time and energy trying to erase without much success. There were so many times I lied and covered up for my mother when she got drunk and did something embarrassing. I used to try to hide her drinking from my brother, father, and friends. There were so many times she didn't remember what had happened the night before, but I always did no matter how much I didn't want to.

Starting when I was about nine years old, when I got home from school, I would clean the house, do the dishes, and try to make everything in the house perfect so when my mom got home she would be happy instead of angry or sad. From a young age, I was doing things no child should be responsible for. I grew up way too quickly. This is why playing and joking around were never easy for me. I was too busy cleaning or trying to protect my brother from what our mother said or did after she had been drinking. I even used to lock my brother in his bedroom and not let him out or stand in front of his door so our mother couldn't get in. It got better for a while when my little sister Eliza was born, but the improvement didn't last. I ended up trying to protect Eliza too even though I was in college by then.

Being the child of an alcoholic is complicated and difficult. You have a skewed vision of what the world is like. Your glasses are most definitely not rose-colored. You are all too aware of the lying, the covering up, and the deceiving. You are all too accustomed to feeling shame, fear, and anger. Especially anger. It comes way too easily. And you believe and think in extremes. There is only black or white, right or wrong, perfection or failure. You go down one of two extreme paths. You either become an alcoholic yourself or you become an overachiever. You don't know you have more than two choices.

I became an overachiever. I protected myself from walking down my mother's path of alcoholism by always pushing harder, doing more, running faster, and working harder than I had to. I made sure I was going to live my life differently than my mother did.

I love my mother. I also know she may not forgive me for putting this in writing, but this is my story to tell. To understand my story, who I am, and what I have been through, you need to know where I came from. I have blanks in my story. I've repressed many parts of my childhood. I simply don't remember a lot of middle school or high school because it was just too much for me to process.

My mom and I have had a rocky relationship over the

years. Sometimes things will be great, and we will laugh so hard together that we start to cry. And then there have been times when we haven't spoken for months and months. I don't always know what version of her I will encounter, and that still scares me even though I'm an adult.

Throughout my life, I've struggled to find ways of coping that were different from my mother's. I've always been afraid that I would end up making the same mistakes she did. This fear drove me to seek other outlets for my feelings of anger, fear, shame, and anxiety. Running was one of the ways I coped with my mother's alcoholism and my feelings about it. When I ran, I didn't have to answer to anyone or explain anything. My high school didn't have a cross-country team, so I didn't need to run because I was in training or competing. I ran because I wanted to run, because I needed to run.

We lived on a hilly dirt road in Vermont. There were lush green mountains on either side, green pastures, and the cleanest air I've ever tasted. There is no pollen or pollution. You can taste how clean it is when you inhale, as the air travels down your throat and fills up your lungs.

Everywhere you turn in Vermont, there is a magnificent view worth stopping to take in. It's a beautiful place to grow up and a beautiful place to run, although I'm not sure how much I was able to appreciate it at the time. In the fall, you're surrounded by brilliant colors on every tree branch. One morning you wake up, and the entire side of the mountain has changed from green to red overnight. The air has new crispness to it that says autumn is here. Then, as the leaves slowly fall one by one, they create a colorful blanket on the ground. The challenge as a runner is, with every step you take, you must negotiate where to place your foot because the ground is different from one day to the next.

The winter is bone-chilling cold — sometimes too cold for it to snow. When it did snow, I would catch snowflakes on my tongue as I ran. I used to see how many I could catch at a time, but it was a bit difficult to keep track while running. The crunching of the snow beneath my feet and being outside when everyone else was bundled up in front of the fire felt liberating to me. I loved running in the snow, especially the morning after a big storm. Making the first tracks in the snow took my breath away. I loved turning around and seeing that my steps were the only ones for miles around. I could run on main roads without seeing a car for twenty minutes or more. The aloneness, the isolation, was exhilarating.

When I got upset, I would throw on my running shoes and sprint out my front door with no idea of where I was going or how long I'd be gone. I would run down the dirt road or into the woods where I could be alone. I ran for miles as fast and as long as I could. Running gave me a sense of freedom and control when I felt like I had none. I ran until I couldn't breathe, tears and dirt streaking down my face. It was my way to deal with and escape what was going on at home.

So was getting caught up in partying with my friends and drinking too much. I was more interested in escaping, in finding a way out, than how I accomplished my escape. In the beginning, I enjoyed partying just as much as running. However, as I got older, running became more and more important to me. When I got to college, it became part of who I was and began to define who I was going to become.

After my parents divorced, my father's coping mechanisms seemed to be endurance exercise and cooking. When my brother and I went to his house on weekends, he would cook recipes from *Bon Appétit* and test them on Luke and me. I always used to say things like, "Gross! I don't want to eat that." I'm sure I would love the recipes now, but when you're in middle school everything with the slightest taste seems gross. Now that I can't run anymore, I find myself also cooking a lot and testing recipes on my family. And sure enough, sometimes I am the one hearing, "Gross! I don't want to eat that!"

My father didn't talk about how much he exercised when we were younger, but we were always around it. I saw pictures of him and his friends from the RAGBRAI cycling event in Iowa and remember thinking, "I want to do that someday." He used to bring us to his friend's house to watch the Tour de France every July, and I would groan, "Do I have to?"

My father would explain to us what each jersey meant and the rules of the race. I can still hear him yelling at the cyclists on television as if they could hear him, coaching them as they climbed. I would watch parts of the race, but most of the time I would try to find friends I could spend time with outside on the porch or in the backyard. And now I host my own Tour de France party every year, every bit as caught up by the race as my father.

Every summer, I accompanied my father and stepmother, Cindy, to a local bike race. I would help man the tent where the cyclists came to pick up their numbers, or we would drive the course to make sure everything was marked so none of the cyclists got lost. I also watched my father when he ran in the Boilermaker 15K Road Race, cheering loudly on the sidelines when he ran by.

I loved hearing stories about my dad running marathons and how fast he was. My goal was to beat his best marathon time someday just so I could say I was faster than he was. We used to joke about it, and he would always say it wasn't going to happen. He was right. I never was able to beat his time, but it wasn't because I didn't have the drive or the ability. It was because my body wouldn't let me push harder — something I didn't understand at the time, but I do now.

One of my favorite stories is about my father running his last marathon without even training for it. He was out with friends one night, having a few beers, and they bet him a case of beer he couldn't run the marathon the next day. He won the bet because he did run the race. He just couldn't walk afterward! Not only did I laugh hearing this story, I also completely understood why he did it. Competition is in my blood just as much as it was in his.

I come from a family of athletes, where everyone has always played sports. My uncles and cousins as well as my brothers, Luke and Joseph, and sister, Eliza, all were involved in some sport. My family was as competitive as it was athletic. There was much talk about this family member setting the local high school basketball record and that family member setting the football record.

The high school I went to in Vermont didn't have enough students for a cross-country or a track and field team. Instead, athletic activities for girls were limited to basketball, soccer, cheerleading, and softball. I did them all. Unlike so many members of my family, I was never good at basketball, but I tried to improve. My incredibly patient Uncle Mike tried so hard to teach me how to play, in his driveway. But I never really got it so eventually I moved on. I liked soccer, but I was never very good at following the playbook.

I loved being a cheerleader in high school even though I kept my past as a cheerleader a secret for a while when I got to college. Every year, we competed in the state championship, and most of the time we won. It was thrilling to hear the crowd cheering and then hear our name called because we had won first place. I was on the varsity team my freshman year in high school, and I was a squad captain my junior and senior years.

I enjoyed being on a team, so I had fun playing softball. I played all through middle school and high school and even made the middle school all-star team. My freshman year in college, I played a little bit, but not for very long. I got too easily sidetracked with college life and wasn't particularly dedicated to softball.

The first semester of my junior year in college, I studied abroad in Australia. I had a wonderful time, but I got into some bad habits. I ate food that wasn't good for me, drank way too much, and even smoked cigarettes. When I got back to the States, I stayed at my father's house over the winter break. At first, I stayed up all night and slept all day because of the time change. Then I just continued that way because that's what I was used to doing in Australia. One day, I finally woke up and decided to get my act together. My father and stepmother had that kind of effect on me. They saw the bad choices I was making and basically gave me the kick in the butt I needed to change course.

I went back to college for the spring semester and slowly started to drop the bad habits I had acquired while I was in Australia. That summer, I decided to live with my father. It would be a summer that would end up shaping the next decade of my life. Throughout high school and college, I had struggled with whether I was going to follow in the footsteps of my mother or go in a different direction. This is a common struggle for children of alcoholics. That summer was when I started to run regularly again. It was also the clear moment in time when I made a very conscious decision not to go down my mother's path. Running played a pivotal role in that decision because it gave me the confidence I needed to change direction and make different choices. I started down my new path by quite literally putting one foot in front of the other and taking one (running) step at a time.

I'm not sure what made me decide to lace up my shoes that first day, but I did. I pulled up to the local park in the middle of town, parked the car, and sat there. I was out of shape because I hadn't run in about a year, and I didn't really want anyone to see me. After several minutes, I told myself, "Okay, Kate. You can't just keep sitting here. It's better to at least try to run. C'mon, you can do this."

I stepped out of my car and onto the sidewalk in the park and just stood there. I was acutely aware of how uncomfortable I was. I wasn't sure what to do next. Should I stretch? Should I walk first? Was I wearing the right clothes? I ended up sitting down on the empty cold sidewalk and stretching a little. There weren't many people out walking because it was early in the afternoon, and most people were still at work. I had chosen what time of day to run quite deliberately. I wanted as few witnesses as possible.

It was a typical cool and breezy upstate New York summer afternoon. The sun was out, but it wasn't humid or hot. It was easy to breathe. The grass was green, and I could hear the wind as it moved through the trees. I love that sound. It's so peaceful and calming.

I started by running a half-mile out and back. The first few steps were exhilarating, the next few more difficult. I could feel the blood rushing to my legs and my heart beating faster than it had in quite some time. Then my legs started to burn, and I had to walk a little. I ran out of breath frequently and had to stop and rest. I remember thinking, "Wow! This is harder than I thought it was going to be!"

But I didn't give up. I kept going until I made it back to the car. I had been so afraid of what people would think of me running so slowly with the wrong shoes and clothes, but no one even noticed me. No one said anything. When I told my father I had gone running that day, all he said was, "Good." I had made myself so anxious about getting back out there and for no reason whatsoever. That night I slept better than I had in a long time.

The next morning I was sore, but I decided to run anyway. It took several weeks, but eventually I was running every day. Each week I added a little more distance and a little more speed. The short one-mile loop turned into two miles, then four, then six.

And I fell head over heels in love with running all over again. I noticed the difference it was making to my body. I lost the fifteen pounds of beer and late-night snacking weight I had gained in college and Australia. I loved that I could see the definition of my calves and quadriceps. My pants felt looser and my shirts felt larger.

I felt more focused and stronger. I started to reassess where I was going in life and how I was going to get there. Things became clearer to me. I started to crave running, and when I missed a day, it really changed my mood. When I ran, I was more energetic and felt happier. Research has indicated that for some people running is like taking an anti-depressant, and that was true for me.

That summer, I started to hang out with runners and become ingrained in the running culture. Runners truly are a different breed. They stick together and encourage and support each other. Things that might offend other people – like shooting snot out of the side of their nose or peeing on the side of the road are considered acceptable behaviors. And they talk about even the most personal things while running. Let's face it. When you spend so much time running, it is easy to get to know each other quickly and on a very personal level.

I ended up dating a physical therapist, and we would frequently run together. When he told me he was planning on running the Boilermaker 15K in July, I thought, "There's no way I can run nearly ten miles!" Little did I know that ten miles would eventually feel like a warm-up to me. However, that summer I watched from the sidelines as Matt crossed the finish line.

The sidelines were full of cheering fans, friends, and family members. There was barely enough space to stand because we were packed in, shoulder to shoulder, standing on our tippy toes to see the runners crossing the finish line. People were holding up signs. "One more mile to the beer." "This was a better idea when you signed up three months ago."

Jets flew over the finish line. There was live music, lots of laughing, and hot, smelly runners everywhere. I became completely caught up in the energy of the runners and the crowd. I could feel the excitement and sense of accomplishment in the air. That was the moment I knew I didn't want to be on the sidelines anymore. After the race, I met Matt and some other friends, and we went to the after-race party. Every moment, I fell more deeply in love with running and the community that comes with it.

The more I ran, the happier I was. I didn't have to think about anything else. Running consumed me. One afternoon, I went on a run with Matt, and he said, "You're fast! Do you realize how fast you are?" His comment felt so good! I had discovered something I was good at that I loved. Matt's words that day only fueled me more and stirred up the competition already bubbling in my blood.

When I got back to college, it was clear that living with Cindy and my father and running had changed me. I had become a different version of myself, one that I really liked. I was athletic, more confident, and determined. I felt good about my body and the direction I was heading in. I felt stronger than I had ever been both physically and mentally.

A few months into the semester, Matt and I broke up. Once

again, running became an escape for me. I had no interest in getting into another relationship, so I ran far and fast, letting my entire world become consumed by running. I decided if Matt could run a 15K, then I could run an even longer distance. If he could run an 8:30 mile, then I could clock an even faster time. I began to regularly run the five-mile loop around my college campus — sometimes once and sometimes twice depending on how I was feeling. I forgot that I was sad or upset about the break-up with Matt. I pushed all my emotions away, and I ran.

I became less and less interested in college parties because I wanted to wake up and run in the morning. I even earned the name of Grandma when I started going to bed at 9:00 or 10:00 pm instead of staying out late on the weekends. Don't get me wrong. I still went out and had fun, but I was more disciplined. I valued running and exercising above drinking and partying. My friends would ask, "Is fun Kate coming out tonight or boring Kate?" What a difference from just a short time before when I had been in Australia! My goals and priorities had shifted and were continuing to shift.

In the fall and winter of my senior year in college, I trained for my first race. In typical Kate fashion, it was a half marathon — a rather ambitious goal for a first race. It made no sense to me to run a shorter distance when I knew I was capable of running 13.1 miles. My competitive nature made me believe that "just" running wasn't enough. Running faster and farther was always better.

The race was the Hyannis Half Marathon, and I stayed with a running friend at her house the night before. I was so nervous and had no idea what to do. She told me she always stretched before going to bed and laid out her race clothes for the morning, so I did too. I even pinned my number onto my shirt so I wouldn't have to fumble with the safety pins in the morning. I lay awake most of the night because I was too excited to sleep.

The sun came up, and it was a snowy and cold day. I had butterflies in my stomach and ate a bagel with peanut butter even though I usually never consumed that kind of food before I ran. Since I had never raced before, I didn't know what I should do. So I kept looking around at all the other runners. Everyone seemed to have a watch, but I didn't. I made a mental note to buy one. Some people were jogging in place, others were huddled up trying to keep warm, and some were stretching. I just stood there and took it all in. The butterflies had moved up to my chest, and I could feel the adrenaline starting to kick in.

The national anthem was played, the gun went off, and the race started! All my training went out the window immediately and, like all novice runners, I went out too fast because I was so excited to be running in a race. I wove in and out around people and up on the sidewalk, wasting precious energy and not even knowing it.

There had been a huge winter storm that week, and the streets were lined with piles of snow that made them narrower than usual. I wore a Turtle Fur neck warmer to help with the cold, and condensation built up around it near my mouth. The little hairs in my nose started to freeze, and then, further into the race, even my eyelashes froze. And I loved it! I loved the crowd yelling and cheering, the exhilaration I felt when I ran past people as they slowed down, the burning and pure exhaustion in my muscles, the pumping of my heart and the rush that gave me.

I ran as fast and as hard as I could that day, with no race plan and no idea what I was doing. About a mile from the finish line, I thought, "I still have a whole mile to go! I don't know if I can do this." I wasn't sure how I was going to keep putting one foot in front of the other because I had gone out so hard, but somehow I did. I finished in 1:46:34. Not too bad for my first half marathon, but I had no idea back then if it was a good or bad time. I waited at the finish line for my friend, and I was bent over and breathing hard. The stiffness didn't take long to set in, and neither did my love of racing.

The best part of it was that I had no idea what I was doing! I didn't know anything about strength training, stretching, ice baths, negative splits, or nutrition. I was a complete mess. Thinking back, I was the perfect example of everything runners do wrong in their first race.

Once I got back to campus that night, I remember thinking how amazing it was that I had run 13.1 miles and had survived! I was so exhausted that 7:30 pm seemed like the perfect bedtime. As the hours went on, I got progressively sorer, and I paid for my lack of racing knowledge for days. I had to go down stairs sideways and winced with each step. My knees were stiff, and it took me a few extra moments to straighten my legs when I stood up. I was completely drained. But none of that mattered because I was so proud of my accomplishment.

From then on, I majored in running. I wanted to know everything about it. How to get better, how to feel good in a race, how to prevent injury, what to eat, what to drink, what shoes to wear, what kind of gear to use. I began to study every single aspect of running I could. I bought books upon books and magazines upon magazines. I read everything I could find online. Then I stepped it up a notch. I began pestering every runner I knew for more information. I was completely and utterly addicted and blissfully in love with running.

2

The Marathon

"Training for and running a marathon is not a single event, rather it is an experience. It is a discovery of self that will forever change your perceptions, perspectives, priorities and possibilities. You will meet yourself at what you thought were the boundaries of your potential and endurance and watch in awe as they evaporate to reveal only an open expanse. To know that the boundaries in life are those, which we create ourselves, is a discovery that cannot be taught — it must be experienced. For once you have seen the view from the mountain — living life of voluntary blindness is no longer an option."

- Sara Mitsch

I graduated from college a year after I completed my first race. I moved to an apartment in Quincy, Massachusetts with two of my college roommates, Allison and Kate. We lived in a great apartment on Pleasant Street, only a short ride on the T (the subway) into Boston. It was the second floor of an old, creaky house, and it was huge. The three of us each had our own room, there was a large kitchen with a lot of windows, and there was an attached screened-in porch. We had a dining room that served primarily as a place to store our extra clothes and iron our outfits in the morning before work. Our living room was also quite large, but the doorways were narrow. We could barely get the plaid sleeper couch and oversized green chair from my father and Cindy into the room. For a long time, we didn't even have a kitchen table or chairs.

The wooden floors creaked wherever we walked throughout the house, and the heat, such as it was, came from old radiators. It was cold in the winter and hot in the summer. The kitchen had wall-to-wall lime-green tiles from the 1950s, and the bathroom sported powder-pink tiles with black-and-white smaller tiles as an accent. Despite the dated color choices and the dated everything, the place was fantastic. I loved my roommates, and I loved having our own place. We were finally grown-ups, even if we had to sit on the kitchen floor to eat!

I had my entire life planned out before I even got my first job. I just knew I was going to love my first job, and I was going to make a ton of money right off the bat. I even pictured myself driving down to Cape Cod on weekends in my Audi A4. My roommate Kate and I shared this dream. She used to say, "A4 by 24!"

Of course, that is not at all how it happened, and I was totally disappointed. Like many people newly graduated from college, I struggled. I was unhappy. I wasn't sure who I was or what I wanted to do with my life. This was not what I had expected being an adult would be like.

Eventually I joined a gym. I walked in on my first day, and I felt very intimidated. I hadn't really lifted weights consistently, and the only gym I'd gone to regularly was the one at college. However, I persevered. Many evenings on my way home from my job, I stopped to work out for a few hours to clear my head. I lifted weights and did yoga. If the weather was lousy and I couldn't run outside, I would run on the treadmill for five to eight miles as fast as I could. I never enjoyed running on the treadmill, so I always tried to get it over with as soon as possible. I was that obnoxious person on the treadmill — the one that looks over to see how fast you are running and then makes sure she is running faster. What can I say? I was competitive, and I was in my twenties.

My first job was not what I had always dreamed it would be. I worked at Chadwicks of Boston, designing and putting together the pages of their catalog. When I was in college, I had done an internship there as well as at a hip advertising firm in the city. Unfortunately, the hip advertising firm wasn't hiring, but Chadwicks was. I needed a job, and my father insisted I have health insurance, so I accepted the offer.

I also think I took it because I liked the people there, and it was easy. But I was so bored, and I dreaded going to work. I often got all my work finished before it was due and then asked my colleagues if they needed help. I spent the rest of the time talking on the phone with Kate or Allison to make plans to go out on the weekend, researching local races, or counting down the hours until I could leave and go for a run.

The more unhappy I became, the more I fell in love with running. I loved everything about it — the escape from my reality it provided, the discipline, the training schedules, the people I met, the competition, and especially the feeling of complete exhaustion after a good hard run. It's safe to say I rarely did anything but a good hard run. An easy run wasn't in my vocabulary. Running really brought out my Type A personality, and it emphasized my perfectionist tendencies and my desire to be completely in control.

My favorite runs were hill repeats and long runs. Hill repeats are runs that focus on running up and down hills over and over again. Sometimes you find a short, steep hill, and other times you find a long, slow hill. Both versions of hill repeats are difficult, but they make you a stronger and fitter runner. Long runs are runs that can be anywhere from eight to twenty-plus miles. Sometimes you run them slowly, and other times you run them at race pace, which is rather fast. Long runs are meant to get your body ready to run long distances efficiently.

No matter what kind of run I was doing, the harder the workout was, the better I felt. After I got home from work or the gym, I went out running for an hour or sometimes more. When I ran, I could forget about my unstimulating job, my non-existent boyfriend, and my life that was falling short of my expectations and my dreams. The more I ran, the more addicted I became to running.

One afternoon after work, I picked up the mail, and right in the middle of the stack of bills and advertisements was a flyer from Team In Training, urging me to join their marathon training program. I read it over and over again as I sat in my Subaru (not the Audi A4 of my dreams), which was parked half on the road and half on the sidewalk outside my apartment. It was a perfect running day, and I had intended to go upstairs and change into my running clothes. Instead I just sat there.

Should I go to the informational meeting to see what Team In Training was all about? My initial thought was, "Yes! Why not?" It was quickly followed by, "No, you can't run a marathon. Are you crazy? That's twice as long as you've ever run before." My mental tug of war continued. "But it's for a good cause, to raise money for the Leukemia & Lymphoma Society. Besides, it's only an informational session. It doesn't mean I have to sign up."

An hour later, still sitting in my car, I made my decision. It was dark by then, and the street lights were starting to blink on one by one. I climbed the stairs to the apartment and didn't say a word to either of my roommates. After all, it was only an informational session, right?

When I went to the meeting the following Thursday night after work, I still hadn't told my roommates, just in case I changed my mind. I walked into a big room with a lot of chairs lined up. Someone was standing in the front of the room, and a few other people were sitting down or making their way to the front of the room. There must have been ten or twelve of us altogether.

As the meeting started, the lights dimmed, and a heart-touching and inspiring video came on. I found myself choking back tears. It made perfect sense to me that I should sign up. I loved running, and my brother was a leukemia survivor. I wanted to raise money for a good cause that was so personal to me, and I was starting to get lonely running by myself all the time. I wanted people to run with.

It didn't take much to convince me. I signed up. But I was so nervous about the commitment I had just made that I nearly ran out of the meeting. When I got home, I told my roommates what I had just done. They were both shocked but supportive.

I began training for my first marathon in January, a cold time of year in New England. The temperatures rarely climb above zero degrees Fahrenheit, and that winter was no different. We ran through snow, ice, and puddles of slush that were nearly a foot deep, but the weather didn't discourage me. I enjoyed training for the marathon. I had coaches, a schedule to follow, and a new group of amazing friends to enjoy.

In fact, training with other people was more fun than I had imagined it would be. We met every Thursday for speed workouts and every Saturday for long runs. I looked forward to those days so much, even though they were physically challenging. On Thursdays after work, we met at the MIT (Massachusetts Institute of Technology) track and ran under the lights as the sun went down.

I had a love-hate relationship with speed workouts. I loved passing people on the track, especially the guys. I loved how I felt when I finished, and I loved the results. But I hated how I felt doing them. In my thank-you letter to the people who sponsored me in the race that year, I wrote, "Speed workouts are like running into a brick wall over and over again as fast and as hard as you can because someone told you it would make you faster. It is pure torture, but hey! If it makes you faster, you better believe I'll do it at least once a week!"

Saturday mornings, we met at 8:00 a.m. in the MIT parking lot. Not quite a year after graduating from college, 8:00 a.m. on a Saturday was still early for me. I stopped at Dunkin' Donuts every one of those Saturday mornings on my way to the track and got a cup of French vanilla coffee. I don't care what anyone says, Dunkin' Donuts coffee tastes the best in Boston. I have had it all over the country, and nothing compares to the Dunkin' Donuts coffee brewed in Boston.

By the time we all got to the parking lot, our coaches Mike and Erin were waiting for us. They told us the route for the day and where the water stations were set up along the way, and then they led us in a dynamic stretching routine. Often people shared their stories about how leukemia had affected them, their family, or people they knew.

Then we were off. I typically was in the front of the group where there were a few of us who ran the same fairly fast pace. But sometimes I would hang back to talk to some of the other runners. Our long runs ranged from eight to twenty miles and were sometimes quite difficult.

We did silly things to keep ourselves busy along the way. Libby was a teacher, and she used to sing sixth-grade camp songs or make us play the alphabet game to get through the last few miles. Some runs we talked for hours about our careers, boyfriends, and lives.

On one seventeen-mile run around the Charles River, I told my friend Kathy that I didn't have a boyfriend and I thought I was ready to have one, but it was always so hard to date. She said, "When you meet the right one, you'll know. It's just easy." This was right after she had met Jeff, the man who went on to become her husband. When I met my husband, Brian, years later, I remembered what Kathy had said on that long run around the Charles. She had been right!

The group of women I met at that time became very good friends of mine quite quickly. Since we were raising money for the Leukemia & Lymphoma Society, we had fundraising events during the week and on weekends that we all went to. Some weekends, we got together to talk, drink wine, or hang out. They were all people I wanted to be around. They were brilliant, fun, and driven. We gave each other advice and were there for each other on and off the road. We supported each other, cheered each other on, and learned from each other.

In Boston, running was a way of life. It was so tightly knit into the culture that you couldn't escape it if you wanted to. If you were a runner living in the area, it was assumed you would eventually try to qualify for the Boston Marathon. If you mentioned the word marathon, people's first reaction was, "Oh, have you run Boston?" Or, "Are you qualifying for Boston?" It was almost as if no other marathons even existed.

I had no idea how much the race transforms the city until I was in the heart of the excitement. April is a month of celebration. There's so much electric energy in the air, and the sense of community is more noticeable. In the weeks leading up to the race, the streets slowly come to life with more and more people sporting their Boston finisher shirts, jackets, or shorts. People begin reminiscing about watching the race or running the race year after year. When you're surrounded by this almost mythical event you have no choice but to want to be part of it, and I was no exception.

The first time I watched the Boston Marathon, I didn't know anyone racing, but I stood on Boylston Street and cheered until my voice was gone. Another year, I watched from the sidewalk in Brookline with my roommates. We had a cooler, chairs, and a blanket that we laid out in the grass. It was a hot day, and the runners were throwing water over their heads as they passed. I noticed as some of them began weaving drunkenly from dehydration as they pushed their bodies farther and farther towards the finish line. I wanted so badly to be out there with them as they ran toward the big CITGO sign that signals the Boston Marathon finish line is close.

During the days of the week I wasn't running with my teammates, I still ran on my own. There was a great long, slow hill with just enough incline near the Boston Common, adjacent to Senator John Kerry's house. I used to run up and down that hill for an hour just to see how many times I could do it before I couldn't take another step. I often wondered if people looked out their windows, speculating about what on earth was wrong with me.

Other days, I would run four miles from my apartment to the gym, work out for a couple of hours, and then run home. I ran through snow banks and ice storms every winter. I ran in the rain and in the sunshine. I ran before the sun came up, in the middle of the day, and after the sun went down. I ran whenever and wherever I could. I am smiling just thinking about it.

As part of our training, Mike and Erin had us run races. I ran the Hyannis Half Marathon, the New Bedford Half Marathon, and the Big Lake Half Marathon that winter and spring. With each race, my times got faster and faster, and I could see the progress of my training. The Big Lake Half Marathon in Alton Bay, New Hampshire on May 8th was the last race I ran before the marathon in San Diego for which we had signed up.

I ran with Libby at Big Lake, and, as usual, we played games along the way as we passed people one by one. We got very close to the finish and realized how well we were doing. We stayed together until the finish line was in sight, and then she kicked into high gear. I was close, but I couldn't stay with her. We finished first and second in the race. I felt so good claiming the prize, even though it was for second place.

June finally came after many miles noted in my training log, many hours of races, and even more hours of group runs and building community. The weather in Boston was nice, and we were finally running in shorts again. Two days before the San Diego Rock and Roll Marathon, I headed to California.

The excitement and anxiety were both palpable in the air. The Saturday before the race, we all attended a pasta dinner put on by Team In Training. We were greeted by cheerleaders, coaches from all over the country, mentors, honored heroes, cancer survivors, friends, and family. As we loaded up on the carbohydrates, we listened to people speak. It was a very emotional night. We were reminded over and over about why we were running.

After dinner, we all headed back to the hotel. My mother sent me flowers, and my former boyfriend Matt called to wish me luck. I felt great. I unpacked my race bag, which was fully equipped with a plastic organizer filled with extra safety pins, salt, GU (a calorie-dense gel runners eat for energy), hair ties, bandages, and much more. My teammates always made fun of how organized I was. Jenn, Kathy, Kristen, and I all got ready together. We laid out our socks, shorts, sneakers, and shoes.

Then we wrote the names of cancer survivors on our jerseys. I wrote my brother Luke's name on mine.

At 4:30 the next morning, our alarms went off. I was sick to my stomach because I was so nervous. We all met in the lobby of the hotel for team pictures and to take a bus to the starting line. Once we were on the bus, my friends Jenn and Sarah started making sock puppets to pass the time. The bus dropped us off a mile from the starting line, and it was a dark, uphill walk. Most of us stopped goofing around and began to get quiet.

Just like my first half marathon, I had woken up with butterflies in my stomach that had moved to my chest by the time I got to the starting line. When the gun went off, I could hear the sound of feet hitting the pavement and watches beeping all around me as we started to run. I could smell the ocean and hear the loud music playing over the cheering of the crowd.

The first mile went by way too quickly. Like every first-time marathoner, I went out too fast. I started with the 3:20 pace group. At every marathon and half marathon there are pace groups. Pace groups are formed by people who have the same time goal in mind in which to finish the race. There are usually one or two people known as the pacers who set the pace that everyone else needs to follow to achieve the time in which they want to finish. The pacer holds a sign with the group's time goal, and runners stick with the group the entire race or as long as they can.

I felt great at the beginning with the 3:20 pace group, not so bad in the middle, and then, when the adrenaline was gone, I struggled. At mile twenty-one, I hit the wall. I had never felt anything like it. I fought with myself physically and mentally to keep taking that next step and the one after that and the one after that.

I felt awful. I was exhausted, I was hot, my feet hurt, and my muscles were getting tighter and tighter by the second. I even debated giving up altogether when I couldn't keep up with the slower pace group to which I had switched. I can still feel the cramping and burning in my muscles as I crested the hills, asking myself, "What am I doing this for?" Then I remembered. The overwhelming excitement from the crowd cheering hit me like a wave. The energy from them and the coaches and the other runners took over and kept me going until I saw the finish line.

As I turned the final corner and started to make my way to the finish, my legs felt like they were going to lock up, but they didn't. I just slowly put one foot in front of the other until I saw the black finish line on the ground approaching. I heard a few teammates off to the right yelling my name. I kept moving, and I crossed the line with my hands high in the air. Crossing that finish line was an amazing experience. I felt so powerful and unstoppable. I had pushed through the doubt and physical pain, and I had kept moving. I looked up at the clock and realized I had missed qualifying for the Boston Marathon by five minutes.

I was exhausted. Bent over and breathing heavily, I saw my teammate Kristen and managed to make my way to her through the crowd of people who had finished. We hugged and congratulated each other, and then we decided right then and there that we would do it again. I dreamed of qualifying for Boston, and I had gotten so close — close enough to light a fire inside me to try again, to run another marathon to see if I could make the cut and qualify. I figured all I needed to do was train harder.

I started marathon running to help raise awareness for cancer and to see what I was made of. I learned a lot about myself, including that I could do more than I thought I could. My new-found community had pulled me out of the unhappy place I had been in, and I was really beginning to enjoy living in Boston and no longer being in college. This amazing group of women with whom I had shared so many cups of coffee, so many long runs, and so many glasses of wine had helped me figure out what I wanted to do with my life, and they would remain my friends even when we no longer lived in the same area and saw each other only rarely.

I made three more attempts to train and qualify for Boston over the next two years that I lived in the area. However, even though I trained on the actual course every year, I never quite made the cut. It would still be a few years before I was able to qualify and return to Boston to run the race.

3

Building My Future

"Life isn't about finding yourself. Life is about creating yourself."

- George Bernard Shaw

Running was the catalyst for my career as a physical therapist. It taught me about community, health, goals, disappointment, and achievement. My running coach Erin was a physical therapist, and I loved her. At every practice, I watched her help people on the side of the track or in the parking lot. I used to walk by her slowly as I was cooling down just to hear what she was telling other runners to do.

On a cold night in January, I was running on the MIT track, and there was snow on the ground. It was cold enough to see my breath every time I exhaled. I had just completed a very difficult speed workout with which I was very satisfied because I had been faster than almost all the men and women out there. I heard my friends and teammates commenting on how fast I was, and I loved it. I was twenty-three years old, and I felt invincible.

That night, I finally got up the courage to ask Erin if I could shadow her at work someday to see what she did. Erin enthusiastically replied, "Of course!" I then began to pick her brain about what PTs actually do. I had experienced a small amount of physical therapy when I had injured my knee after my first half marathon in college. I hate to admit it, but I wasn't a good patient. I did only some of the exercises, and I forgot some of my appointments. I would run to and from physical therapy even when my PT had told me not to. In short, I was the patient I would never want to treat!

A few weeks after I had approached Erin, I found myself at her small private practice outside Boston. The clinic was filled with rows of PT tables or plinths crammed into one room. There wasn't much space between or around the tables, and all the exercise equipment was in the front of the room.

Even though it was cramped and small, I felt right at home as I observed Erin treat a few patients. If I was serious about going to school for physical therapy, she suggested I reach out to her friend Jessica for a PT aide job. In order to apply to and get into PT school, you have to have logged several hundred hours of observation, and this was one way to get my hours while making sure I really liked physical therapy. I called Jessica, was interviewed, and got the job. I was ecstatic to be able to quit my job at Chadwicks and start working as a PT aide.

After several months, I ended up moving in with Alexis, one of my coworkers. We lived in Inman Square in Cambridge, only a few short miles from the Charles River and a great place to live. It was easy to get around the city walking, running, or taking the T. There was a great Indian restaurant right around the corner that we loved. We often walked over, bundled up from the cold. We'd laugh out loud at the Bollywood music videos that were always playing in the restaurant then spend a couple of hours eating great Indian food.

Alexis and I created similar work schedules and took turns driving into work and packing each other's lunches. We goofed around and sang in the car on the way into the office, camped out in our living room, and ran together. Alexis helped me with the anatomy classes I was taking at night and talked me through some of the physiology I had a difficult time with.

When I first met Alexis, I wasn't a morning exerciser, and she was. When our alarms went off, she would bounce out of bed, and I would crawl. I hated waking up at 5:00 am to run, but she always seemed so happy to do it. Eventually we both made it out the door. I slowly became accustomed to getting up early, and Alexis became accustomed to my complaining about it!

Despite my grumbling, those morning runs were a lot of fun. We ran and talked and planned our weekends and figured out our lunches for the week. Not only did we run, but we also went to the gym to do spin classes and lift weights. We rode our mountain bikes outside the city on the weekends.

When we first started mountain biking, I was scared. But once I got going, I enjoyed it. I looked forward to our Saturday or often Sunday morning rides when we could get out of the city and be in nature, away from the concrete. We packed food and a couple of gallons of water and drove north. We got covered in mud, riding the trails and laughing so hard our stomachs hurt. Alexis would have to stop when I fell and had to climb back on my bike. It happened frequently, but I never got really injured.

My job as a physical therapy aide at Spaulding Framingham was located about twenty miles outside Boston and coincidentally was also close to the Boston Marathon course. I loved working there. I instantly became friends with a lot of the physical therapists as well as the support staff. I loved the environment, working with athletes, and collaborating with the PTs.

I was learning so much about physical therapy both in and out of the office. PTs in general are quite active, healthy people, and I loved being part of such a group. I eventually convinced many of the PTs I worked with and my running friends from Team In Training to create a team and do the Reach the Beach Relay race in New Hampshire. It is a 212-mile, 24-hour relay race from Bretton Woods Ski Area to Hampton Beach State Park.

I was the team captain and assigned each runner specific legs of the race, based on their ability. We rented two twelve-person white vans to move us along the course, packed a lot of food, water, and supplies, and started off. The weather was typically questionable, and someone always had to run the legs in the woods in the middle of the night with their headlamps on.

We had so much fun that we did it multiple years in a row, and my teammates continued even after I moved to Atlanta. Our team was called Who Sat on My Sandwich. It came from one of the long days or nights (they all blend together on those trips) when we were all packed into one of the vans and someone sat on Jamie's sandwich. It was a silly name for our team, but it made us laugh.

I wasn't making much money working as an aide at Spaulding, and I needed money to go back to school. I was taking prerequisite classes at night after work one or two days a week. So I picked up a waitressing job at a Mexican restaurant on weekends and some week nights. Some evenings, after I got home from work, I would have an hour or so, and then I would have to drag myself into the restaurant. Once I got going, I was usually fine and had plenty of energy, but it was a long day, getting up at 5:00 am and going to bed after midnight. However, because I had finally found what I wanted to do, it didn't really bother me. I had never minded working hard for what I wanted to achieve, and I wanted to be a physical therapist. I was very focused, even if very tired from working two jobs and going to school. But it was all worth it. Once Erin inspired me, I never looked back.

After my prerequisites were finished, I started applying to PT schools. My high school friend Scott was at Georgia Tech and Emory doing an MD/PhD program and suggested I look into Emory. One of my colleagues and teammates from the Reach the Beach Relay, Derek, was an Emory alumnus. He raved about Atlanta and the school and even wrote me a recommendation letter. I ended up visiting Emory in January, and I fell in love with the warm winter weather and the sunshine. I enjoyed the people I met when I toured the school and was in awe of how beautiful the campus was. Many of the buildings on Emory's campus are made of marble and have red tile roofs. The Quad is green, even in January — a far cry from the streets of Boston in January! I ended up applying to Emory, the MGH Institute of Health Professions in Boston, and a few other schools.

I didn't want to leave Boston. I loved the city and my life there. However, I wasn't accepted by MGH, and I was accepted by Emory. So I had to leave if I wanted to go to school, and, even though I was sad, I knew it was the right thing to do. In June, I packed up my Subaru, promised my friends I'd be back right after graduation from Emory, said goodbye to Boston, and headed to Atlanta.

Prior to leaving, I had sold or given away all my furniture and the things I didn't really need because I had no money and no way to bring it all with me. I decided I would buy what I needed when I arrived in Atlanta. I only kept my clothes, some books, and of course all my sports gear. My mountain bike was mounted on the roof rack, and the car was packed floor to ceiling, window to window, with just enough room for my former roommate Kate to drive down with me.

The whole way we laughed, cried, and joked about what would happen next. We took pictures at every state line, even though it meant we had to illegally park on the highway in front of each sign. Living up north, we weren't accustomed to so much open space between cities and couldn't believe it when there was no Starbucks nearby. Several hours north of Atlanta, after stopping at a very scary gas station, we both started to question if I was doing the right thing by leaving Boston to live in the south.

When we arrived, I found out my apartment wouldn't be ready for another night. So we ended up staying with my childhood friend Tom. The next day, we had a good time while Kate helped me move in, and then it was time to take her to the airport to fly home. I was so sad for her to leave and unsure of what the next chapter of my life would look like. The apartment felt so empty and quiet, when I got back from the airport. I wandered around the empty rooms, trying to decide what to do. I didn't have any furniture, not even a bed. I called Scott and asked for help. He had friends with an extra mattress and box spring and even an extra coffee pot. A lifesaver! Now I had everything I needed.

The following day, my new roommate, Lori, whom I had met at orientation, arrived. We signed up and ran a 10K the first month we were at Emory, where we both won first in our age groups, and we had a wonderful time at the race. It was nice to have a roommate to run with right off the bat. I was less lonely but still longing for my life back in Boston.

Like-minded people once again surrounded me in PT school. Many of my classmates ran, were cyclists, lifted weights, camped, or were very active, which was no surprise. It's very beneficial for a physical therapist to be active because the job is so physical. The job also entails educating patients about health, wellness, and exercise. So being active not only allows a PT to relate to their patients, but also gives the physical therapist credibility as someone who walks the talk.

PT school was difficult. I needed to do a lot of studying that entailed many late nights. I loved what I was learning, but I struggled sometimes. I had never really had to study before, so

I had to learn good study habits in graduate school. I often fell asleep, drooling, in the library. So I found myself studying at coffee shops a lot.

I would bring my stacks of books, get a coffee or two, put on my earphones, and sit cross-legged and barefoot in my chair, studying for hours. I had so many books, notecards, and highlighters that it was common for books to start falling off the table. When I got looks from the other coffee shop patrons, I didn't know if it was because of the loud music I was listening to or the loud noises my books were making!

About six months after moving to Atlanta I met Brian, my husband. One night I went out with some of my friends from school to celebrate their birthdays. When my friends and I arrived at the bar Brian was sitting alone at one of the small tables outside, waiting for someone. My friends and I wanted a picture of all of us, so I walked up to Brain and asked him if he could take it. I was the designated driver that night, as I had a race coming up in a couple weeks. However, I sat at the bar all night with Brain laughing, talking about marathon running, and debating politics. That was it. I was done. From that night on we became inseparable whenever he was in town. His job required him to travel a lot, which was okay for us at that point in our lives. I had plenty of time for school, studying, friends, and running.

I continued to run a lot and train for races while in school. It was a great way to relax and get outside after being trapped indoors, staring out the window at the beautiful weather while studying for hours. I ended up starting a running group and created track workouts, training schedules, and hill repeat workouts for my friends. I didn't mind writing up the workouts because I was glad to have people to run with again. The group of us would sign up for half marathons or marathons and travel to the race together or, if the race was in Atlanta, meet very early in the morning to go together. It was a lot of fun.

During training, we made sure to meet once or twice a week to do workouts together. I usually wrote up the workouts a week ahead of time, and then everyone would meet at the track and get started. There was a hill just off Emory's campus that we would run to from the track. It was just long enough and steep enough to make everyone complain a little bit. As we ran up and down, we would cheer each other on, and most people were relieved when that part of the workout was over. Other nights, we would sprint around the track, doing four-hundred-, eight-hundred-, or sixteen-hundred-meter sprints.

Eventually, my friend Lindsay convinced me we should do a triathlon. I thought, "Why not?" I had been running so much, and my last marathon, the Philadelphia Marathon, hadn't gone very well. I needed a change of pace and some variation in my workouts, so triathlon seemed like a great idea. There was something very appealing to me about doing three sports instead of one in the same race!

As I was training for my first triathlon, I was also training for the Columbus Marathon. I wrote the running training schedule for the triathlon, and Lindsay helped me train for the cycling and swimming components. We helped each other. I ended up really enjoying the addition of cycling and swimming to my routine. I wasn't a good swimmer, but I wasn't sinking either! Some afternoons after class or between classes, we would sneak in a swim, a bike, or a run. Sometimes, if we didn't have enough time, we would grab a couple of spin bikes at the gym, and we would have our own class with Lindsay as the spin instructor.

It was Lindsay who taught me about bricks, how to set up your transition area, how to swim more efficiently, and basically everything I didn't know about triathlon, which was a lot. A brick workout is a workout that consists of two disciplines performed back to back. For instance, you might ride a bike for an hour then jump off the bike, change your shoes, and begin running. The first day I ever did a brick, I thought my legs were going to buckle. I quickly realized the workouts were called bricks because your legs feel as heavy as bricks. The first few steps coming off the bike are the most difficult, but after a few minutes your legs start turning over more easily.

Transitions are exactly what they sound like, the transition from one discipline in the triathlon to the next. I learned that becoming efficient in your transitions saves you time and agony later in the race.

I didn't have a road bike or triathlon bike and certainly didn't have any money in graduate school to buy one, so I trained and competed on my mountain bike. I thought nothing of it because I didn't know any better. Mountain bikes are heavy and have wide tires. They are neither efficient, nor fast, nor comfortable to ride when doing a triathlon, but I didn't care. I could still feel the wind on my face as I pedaled forward.

Lindsay and I did the Sunbelt Cohutta Springs Triathlon in October 2007. The race was a half-mile swim, an eighteen-mile bike ride, and a four-mile run. I was nervous but not nearly as nervous as when I ran my first half marathon because this time

I knew I was better prepared. I had trained well, had a race plan, and, since I'd been running marathons, a sprint triathlon didn't seem like a big deal.

The race was just over a two-hour drive north of Atlanta. We decided to get up very early in the morning and drive to it in Lindsay's SUV, which could hold our bikes, helmets, running shoes, goggles, swimsuits, race bags, and plenty of food. It was still dark when we left Atlanta, and there was no one on the highway. When we arrived, we were very early but were able to set up our transition area. I watched what Lindsay did and followed suit. I put a towel on the ground, laid out my socks, shoes, shorts, sunglasses, and helmet. We set our bikes up at the end of the row in order to get in and out of the transition area faster. Then we went back to the car to sleep for a little while.

Our alarm went off just as the sun started to come up. The once-quiet field we had parked in was now full of people getting ready for the race. All around us, people were getting their bikes out, changing into their race gear, checking the air in their tires, putting sunscreen on, warming up, and heading to check-in. Lindsay and I got out of the car and went to get officially checked in.

In a marathon, you only have one number to deal with, but in triathlon you have at least three — one for your helmet, one for your bike, and one for the run — plus a timing chip to wear on your left ankle. Then you go through a body-marking station typically located near the entrance of the transition area. Volunteers write your race number in sharpie on both of your arms and calves as well as your age on the back of your left calf. There is something strangely calming about going through the check-in process. Once you have set everything up and your body is marked, you know you are ready.

I was most worried about the swim portion of the race. I knew I could do it, but I also knew I wasn't a very good swimmer. I couldn't wait to be done with that part. About twenty minutes before the race began, Lindsay and I were waiting on the shore of the mucky, dirty lake. We stood there in our swimsuits, Velcro straps around our ankles with our timing chips on them, bodies marked, swim caps and goggles in hand. She reminded me to take my time and stay on the outside of the group to avoid getting kicked in the head or swum over.

The race started in waves. I saw the first wave go, and then, when the loud horn went off for my wave, I was momentarily paralyzed. Then I ran in with everyone else and stayed to the left. It was chaos! Legs and arms were flying everywhere. I had a difficult time catching my breath at first and had to calm myself down. I did get kicked, swallowed water, and even started to swim in the wrong direction at one point, but I made it. When I finally ran out of the water, I was so relieved.

I ran to my bike, threw shorts on over my bathing suit, dried off my feet, and ran out of the transition area with my bike. The weather was perfect. It was sunny, but not too warm, and there was a breeze.

Lindsay had passed me in the water as I had expected, but I was determined to catch her on the bike. If I had realized what a disadvantage I was at on my mountain bike, I probably wouldn't have tried. But I was so naïve and there was so much excitement and adrenaline coursing through my body that I worked very hard to catch up to her. Several seasoned triathletes passed me, saying encouraging things like, "Wow! You are killing it on a mountain bike," and "Great job! You're almost there." It was abundantly obvious that I was a newbie, but I did manage to catch Lindsay a few miles from the last transition area.

My legs were surprisingly more tired than I expected in my first four hundred meters of the run. However, with each step I was less awkward and more in my element. I was invigorated by everything I had already accomplished. The closer I got to the finish, the more excited I became. At the finish line, people were cheering loudly, and there was so much energy and excitement.

I finished, and a few minutes later Lindsay crossed the finish line too. I was sold! I was no longer a runner, but an endurance athlete. For the next several weeks I proudly wore my triathlon T-shirt and told everyone how much fun it was.

Three weeks later Brian and I went to Ohio to run the Columbus Marathon. He had intended to run the full marathon but hadn't been able to train well because of his work schedule. So he ended up running the half marathon, and I ran the full one. This time, I was determined to qualify for Boston!

As usual, I was nervous at the starting line but settled in rather quickly and stuck with my pace group. The triathlon training served me well. I was stronger and better than I had been in any other race, and I was actually enjoying myself. Around mile twenty-two, Brian jumped in and ran most of the remaining 4.2 miles with me. The closer to the finish line I got, the more excited and nervous I became. I was on pace to qualify! Brian reminded me to slow down and stay calm, because the last race I had been so close and then had blown it at the finish. I listened to him and finished in 3:38:57, qualifying for my first Boston Marathon!

That summer, I moved to Birmingham, Alabama for six months to do two of my three clinical rotations required in PT school. I wasn't excited to go to Birmingham, my only knowledge of it being what I had learned in school about the civil rights movement. When I first arrived, I was staying in the UAB (University of Alabama at Birmingham) dorms. It wasn't the best area, and I really didn't know anyone, so I started to feel a little depressed. Then, thankfully, two amazing things happened. First, my friend Meg from PT school put me in contact with her Aunt Katheryn and Uncle Brad. They were unbelievable. They invited me to move in with them, to their house in Mountain Brook, for nearly five months, and it made a world of difference. Then my clinical advisor, Lisa, introduced me to a little running store in Homewood called the Trak Shack. That was all I needed to fall in love with Birmingham.

It was so easy to meet fellow runners, and within a few days I found myself a new running partner, Natalie. She had just qualified for the Boston Marathon too, and we had the same pace and drive, and a lot to talk about! We became friends immediately. Running was really helping me settle into my new community, and I quickly became part of it. I now look back at Birmingham as one of my favorite memories of PT school.

Natalie and I trained for the Boston Marathon week after week, month after month. We met at the Trak Shack on weekends to do our long runs, we got up early before work to do track workouts, and we met any other day of the week we could to train, run together, and just hang out.

Birmingham is hot and humid. There were morning and evening runs when I could taste the salt running down my face and feel the sweat burning my eyes. We kept moving our runs earlier and earlier in the morning to avoid the humidity, but no matter what time you run between March and September in Birmingham, it is nearly unbearable. So we settled on 4:45 am two days a week and just sucked it up.

In April 2009, we ran our first Boston Marathon! It was everything and more than I could have hoped for. I had run so many races, that running a marathon wasn't such a big deal anymore. However, running the Boston Marathon was a huge deal. Brian, my father, my stepmother, and my little brother Joseph all came to Boston to cheer me on. I felt overwhelmed by the opportunity and the love all around me.

Most runners take school buses from downtown Boston to Athletes' Village in Hopkinton, but there was an Atlanta running group that had a charter bus, and Natalie and I were lucky enough to get two seats on it. The bus was temperature-controlled and had a bathroom. Having an easily accessible bathroom before a race is a luxury!

As we pulled away, I watched out the window and waved goodbye to Brian. The ride to Athletes' Village was full of excitement and promise. The weather was warm, but nothing compared to Birmingham. As we drove, I watched as we passed school bus after school bus of other runners heading to the very same place. When the bus pulled up to drop us off, I began to get my typical butterflies. I was thinking about every marathon I had run to get here, and now I was finally here!

A band was playing music up on a stage, and there were several event tents to sit under, porta potties, and people everywhere. Photographers wandered the village, taking pictures of runners as they lay on the ground stretching, sleeping, or drinking their coffee.

Boston is unlike any other marathon for so many reasons. For one thing, the race itself starts later in the day than most marathons, so there is time to lounge around beforehand and obsess about the upcoming race. Athletes' Village is essentially a holding ground for all the athletes during that time.

When it got close to the race start, Natalie and I made one last stop at the porta potty and jogged toward our starting corral. The streets were overtaken with runners. People sat on sidewalks, climbed over fences, and hung out on lawns — all in anticipation of the gun going off. We stood in our corral, waiting for what seemed like a very long time. The National Anthem came and went. And then the gun went off!

Natalie and I decided that we had worked so hard to qualify and train for Boston that we were going to take it all in and enjoy ourselves. The first several miles of the course are downhill, so it is easy to get caught up in the excitement and go out too fast. Luckily for us, we had planned on taking it easy, so we took pictures of signs along the way, talked, and laughed, just like we had during every long run we had done together before.

Since I had lived in Boston previously, many of my local friends lined various parts of the course to cheer me on. Around mile eighteen, Alexis was watching the race with some of my other friends from Spaulding. My knee was bothering me a little, so she spent some time stretching me out and doing a little soft tissue work on it before I got into all the hills.

Once we made it through the Newton hills and were heading into Boston, we saw the famous CITGO sign. I got a little emotional and started to tear up. I had watched so many other runners at this part of the race in years past, and now it was my turn! As we approached Boylston Street, the excitement in the air built and built and built. The noise from the crowd got louder and louder and louder.

When we turned the corner, I heard my name. My best friends from college, Kate, Allison and Sarah, were there holding up signs of encouragement and watching me run by. The streets were lined with people three to five deep. Running down Boylston is like running down a loud tunnel of clapping, cheering, and excitement that pushes you toward the finish line. No other race experience comes even close.

Around four hours after leaving Hopkinton, Natalie and I crossed the finish line. It was the first race I had run where I was more energized than exhausted. My family was waiting at the finish line to give me congratulatory hugs and kisses, and my friends had secured a spot at a nearby bar for the post-race celebration. I couldn't wait to rehash the entire race with every friend, family member, or person I saw who was willing (or unwilling!) to listen.

I was so proud of qualifying for and running the Boston Marathon that I wore my medal to class the next week and showed everyone who cared and many who didn't. My nana and grandmother cut out the results in the local newspapers and sent them to me. I had achieved exactly what I had hoped for, and I had loved every single minute. I couldn't wait to do it again and again and again.

4

Too Many Bad Days

"In questions of science, the authority of a thousand is not worth the humble reasoning of a single individual."

- Galileo Galilei

I had run a total of thirteen marathons and three Bostons, and I had completed both sprint and Olympic triathlons. I planned on completing at least one half and one full Ironman, and I wanted to run a 50K I believe I would have achieved these goals and many others I would have set for myself. However, these unmet goals will remain unmet for me.

All athletes have bad days or bad races, but I had too many. Of my thirteen marathons, I had three very bad days. In three marathons, I passed out and was lucky I woke up. Of course, when it was happening, I didn't see it that way. There was nothing lucky about what was going on. I thought they were simply bad days. I assumed I had pushed myself hard enough to see exactly what I was made of. Which never seemed to be enough.

After each bad day, I told myself I must not be mentally strong enough and that I gave up too soon. I told myself I needed to train harder and be more focused. I beat myself up over and over. I replayed each race and the preparation for each race over and over again in my head like a movie trailer, to see if I could find the answer to what had gone wrong. This is how an athlete thinks. This is how we improve. This is how we live. And I was an athlete.

But I could never figure out what had gone wrong. Did I get enough sleep? Did I drink enough water? Was I over-trained or under-trained? Did I go out too fast or too slow? I thought I knew how to train and how to race, but I still kept having issues. I couldn't pinpoint the problem, no matter how many times I went over the data and replayed the day.

However, there was a pattern. In all three marathons in which I passed out, I ran under a lot of stress, during a period of change in my life, and I was pushing myself to go faster or harder. There is a lot of research to support that stress can negatively affect a person's heart rate, breathing, and overall body systems. Those races were the perfect collision of extreme physical and mental stress. In all three of them, I even questioned whether I should run but, regardless of my intuition, I ran anyway. It's simply not in my nature to back out or quit. I have always been the one to achieve, to win, to keep pushing no matter what.

Shortly after I had been accepted into the Emory physical therapy program and as I was getting ready to move to Atlanta, I ran the Vermont City Marathon in Burlington, Vermont.

At that point, I had lived in Boston for seven years and was moving in less than a month. I was incredibly excited about the next step in my life, but I was also nervous about making such a huge change.

It was hot out that day, even before the race started. You could feel the humidity building in the air as the sun started to come up. I was under a lot of emotional and mental stress. I wanted so badly to qualify for Boston since I had been so close the year before. My training had been pretty good, so I thought it was a possibility. Before the race began, I had a sick feeling in my stomach. Not my usual butterflies, something different. For a fleeting moment I wondered if I should pull out of the race, but I didn't.

I started running with my friend Sarah. She had also run the San Diego Marathon with me the year before. At mile two, I knew it wasn't going to be a good day, but I tried to push myself through. As I ran through the cobblestones of downtown Burlington, I asked myself, "Why am I doing this?" Sarah stuck with me for several miles, but I wasn't feeling good, and I told her to go ahead. Each neighborhood I ran through, enthusiastic spectators cheered me on. I kept pushing, even as the heat started to take its toll.

At mile twenty-three, things were a little blurry, and I started to get confused. I could see the green trees around me and feel the pavement under my feet, but I wasn't exactly sure where I was in the race. I began weaving all over the course. I bumped into a few people, before I was pulled to the side of the course by a medic. He wanted to take me in the ambulance, but I refused. I could see the ambulance parked on the side of the road, and I was not getting in it. I didn't care how bad I felt or looked, I was not getting in! I have never been very pleasant under stress and even less so when I'm told I can't do something I know I can do. That day I refused to get into the ambulance, and I refused to stop racing. I was beyond difficult. Now that I am on the other side and treat athletes at races, it seems so ridiculous. Why would you risk your health for a finisher's medal? But, without realizing the impact and risk, that's exactly what I did that day in Burlington.

The medics stayed with me and kept me by the side of the road, giving me food and fluid for nearly an hour. As I lay there, I could feel the anger and frustration seeping into my veins. I knew there was no way I would be qualifying for Boston now. After a while I was no longer dizzy and felt fine. So I fought the medics to get back on the course. I wanted to finish the race no matter what.

I walked and ran the remainder of the race while a medic rode his bike next to me until the finish line was in sight. I cried the whole way. I was angry with myself. I was frustrated that, after so many quality training sessions and so much hard work, my performance was sub-par. I assumed that I hadn't trained properly or had gone out too fast. I felt like I should have known better. I couldn't believe how bad my time was, and I was so embarrassed.

This was the first race my parents had come to see me run. My whole family was there — my mother, stepfather, father, stepmother, grandmother, grandfather, brother, aunt, and uncle. I saw my dad at the finish line and, when he met me, I collapsed into his arms. He picked me up and carried me out of the shoot.

I felt like a child again and wanted to do nothing more than cry. I felt terrible. I thought, "This is what a bad day feels like."

Everyone told me it was okay and that bad days happen. I never followed up with a doctor because everyone around me, including my running friends, told me it was probably dehydration because of the heat. It was eighty-six degrees that day, outrageously hot for Vermont. I didn't know any better at the time, so I told myself that next time I had to train harder and be more prepared.

A year later, I ran the Philadelphia Marathon. It was my first year at Emory, and I was exhausted and stressed out. I had just finished exams, and I hadn't been sleeping well. My college roommate Kate was in Philadelphia studying for her graduate degree. She was going to run the half, and I was running the full because I was still trying to qualify for Boston. Going into the race, I was more nervous than usual because of the pressure I was putting on myself to do well.

I loved the course. It was scenic, flat, and had a lot of support along the way. The temperature was in the fifties, so it was absolutely perfect for me. I felt great for most of the race and was even able to stay with the 3:40 pace group without difficulty.

Then, without warning, I blacked out at mile twenty-six. I saw the finish line, realized I was about to qualify, and then I lost control of my bladder, got dizzy, and started to feel terrible. I woke up, but it took me a while to come to and realize I was in the medical tent. I was scared and completely confused. I was lying on a pea-green Army cot with cold towels in my armpits, no shoes on, and hooked up to an EKG machine. There were a lot of people around me, rushing back and forth. I tried to sit up and pull off the leads, but the doctors gently pushed me back down. I am not sure how long I was in the tent. Eventually Kate came in and sat with me, but I was confused for several hours.

I had no idea if I had even crossed the finish line. I didn't find out until later, when the race results were posted online. When Kate and I were back in her room, we went online and checked for the results over and over until we saw that I had crossed the finish line. I was so excited and relieved that I had finished. I didn't want to have to explain to anyone why I didn't finish. The strangest thing was that, not only was my time posted, but there were also pictures of me crossing the finish line with my arms above my head celebrating. From the pictures, you would never know I had passed out. I looked completely fine.

Then, as I stared at the images on the screen, I remembered being picked up under my armpits by two other runners a few yards from the finish. I wasn't sure if I had fallen and they had picked me up or if they had caught me. Someone whispered in my ear, "You have to cross the finish line on your feet, by yourself, or it doesn't count." Sitting at the computer, I looked down and saw my skinned elbows and knees. I felt the bruise on my face. I shrugged the whole experience off as being dehydrated. I had no idea at the time how unusual and how lucky it was that I had regained consciousness.

The week after the race, I followed up with a cardiologist at the Emory student clinic as instructed by the doctors in the medical tent. I was nervous, but I didn't think they would find anything. They asked me why I was there since I was "so healthy." I told them I wasn't sure, but the people in the medical tent at the Philadelphia Marathon had thought I should come, so I had.

I was given a stress test, an echocardiogram, and an EKG at the clinic, and none of the tests indicated anything negative. They said nothing was wrong with me and cleared me to go back to my normal life. It was a fluke I had passed out in Philadelphia. I think I ran that very day and thought nothing else of the situation. I assumed I was okay since the cardiologist said I was. I had no reason to believe otherwise.

I continued to run and exercise for four years. I finished physical therapy school. Then Brian and I moved to Chicago so that I could pursue an orthopedic residency. We loved living in Chicago. We lived in a small condo on Lake Michigan and had access to several running trails throughout the city. We ran in the snow, the wind, and cold. One of the offices I worked in was right downtown, so I built my schedule so that I would have two hours in the middle of the day to run around the lake. I loved living and running in Chicago. While Brian and I lived there we ran the Chicago Marathon. I had run it with an injured back, so my time hadn't been very good.

The following year I ran the Chicago Marathon for the second time. I wanted to run it again to prove that I could run faster on the supposedly fast and flat course. At this point, I had already qualified for Boston. So I had faster, more difficult goals in mind. I still wanted to beat my best time and get closer to my father's personal record.

I had just finished my orthopedic residency for physical therapy and had moved back from Chicago to Atlanta. I had started my first official job a few months earlier, and I was just getting over a cold. This time Brian was running the race too. We started out together, but he wasn't feeling well and I was feeling really good. So he told me to go ahead, and I did.

I was running at a good pace, and then suddenly, at mile nineteen, I felt like I needed to sit down. I started to feel anxious, and I slowly made my way to the side of the road where there was a curb. I sat down, and the next thing I knew, I woke up with my feet raised above my head, and there was a police officer with me. He was on his walkie-talkie, calling an ambulance. I wondered who it was for. I was confused and scared again. As fate would have it, the moment I opened my eyes, I saw Brian run by. I yelled out to him, and he heard me. In the middle of hundreds of people, he actually heard me!

I was lying on the ground, and the medics and Brian wanted me to get into the ambulance. They did their best to convince me, but I wasn't having it. I wanted to finish the race. As usual, I was stubborn and refused. Then Brian stepped in and told me, "Get in the ambulance right now," in a voice I had never heard him use before. It was enough to finally make me listen and comply.

Once I was in the ambulance and feeling better, I asked if I could get out of the ambulance and run again. By the looks on their faces, I knew they all thought I was crazy, but I was completely serious. The answer was a resounding "No!"

I ended up in the ER at the University of Chicago Hospital. Several physicians came in to check on me, and five bags of fluid later, they told me I was dehydrated and sent me home. They didn't believe I needed to follow up with anyone. They told me I was fine.

Through the several years I trained and competed, there were many other times that I felt lightheaded or had to stop running because I "felt funny." I never really thought anything was wrong. I always told myself it was the heat, or I was tired, or I hadn't trained enough. I would feel a fluttering in my chest, or I couldn't quite focus. Sometimes I would be running and have to crouch down in the road because something wasn't right, but it would pass, and I'd get right back up. If I was running with a group or a running partner, I was always embarrassed.

Once, when my husband and I were training for a marathon, I suddenly felt lightheaded and dizzy. We were somewhere between miles twelve and fourteen and had several miles left to go. I crouched down and walked a few minutes. Brian gave me some fluid, and I had a GU. After a little while, the feeling passed, and we ended up finishing the twenty-mile run.

That feeling would come and go over the years. In the beginning, it came on infrequently. However, as the years passed, it began to happen more often and last longer. I trained and ran some marathons with no difficulty, but others were disasters. I consistently attributed what happened to being out of shape or just having had a baby or being under-trained. I always had an answer for why I felt poorly.

I never considered the possibility of something else going on. I was young and healthy, and I felt invincible. How could something be wrong? Even though I didn't think it was serious, I did begin to wonder if I should stop running marathons. I told myself I would stop after I had run ten marathons, but I changed my mind. What was the harm in running a couple more?

As if passing out on three occasions wasn't enough, I also had ventricular tachycardia (VT) on three occasions. VT occurs when the electrical system of the heart is no longer doing what it is supposed to do. There are several reasons for someone to go into VT, but it is dangerous. Your heart rate can go unbelievably high, and your rhythm becomes dangerously irregular. So, even though your heart is pumping at a very fast rate, you aren't getting the blood and oxygen you need because the pumping is irregular.

When I was in VT, I should have realized that something was seriously wrong, but I didn't know what was happening. Initially I chose to ignore it because I had already been told I was fine. I thought what I was experiencing was all in my head. It turned out that my symptoms were real, but my belief I was fine was all in my head.

The first episode of VT was about six months before I got pregnant. I had gotten burned out from doing so many marathons and going through PT school and residency. So I had taken some time off from running and triathlon to just coach and chill out, and I was in the process of getting back into shape. That day it was too hot and humid to be running outside, so I went to the YMCA. My friend Jenn and I had just decided we wanted to start training for a half Ironman, so I thought I would start by doing speed work on the treadmill to test where my fitness was.

When I got on treadmills at the gym, I was frequently doing sprints. The harder I pushed myself, the better and more invincible I felt. On this particular day, the gym was packed, but there were a few open treadmills, and the fans were blowing on us to keep the room cool. I was pushing myself very hard. There was a guy in his twenties to my left running 8:00-minute miles and a woman about my age to my right running more slowly. I started off running 8:00 to 8:30-minute miles, but eventually I started doing repeats at 6:50, 6:45, and 6:30 minutes per mile. I loved the feeling of trying to outrun the treadmill.

Then I slowed down and stopped. I immediately felt lightheaded and nervous. I stepped off the treadmill and made my way through the gym quickly. I couldn't get out of there fast enough. By the time I made it outside to the parking lot, my heart was pounding hard, and I wasn't thinking clearly. I paced in circles breathing and trying to slow down my heart rate. I kept thinking, "I just need to calm down." I was so hot. I kept walking up and down the street outside the gym, just pacing. It took several agonizing minutes for my heart rate to finally slow down.

I was scared but not scared enough. I sat in my car for a little while, not sure what to do. After what seemed like an eternity, I decided I was fine. I talked myself into thinking there was no reason for me to be worried. I didn't mention it to anyone, and I went home. Once again, I assumed that I was really out of shape and needed to work harder and put more time into my training.

I continued to train, but then I got pregnant. So I stopped training for triathlon, decreased the intensity of my workouts, and kept running. I slowed down quite a bit and kept my mileage under fourteen miles. Every run I went on after that was to prevent morning sickness rather than to prove to myself how fast I could go! If I hadn't gotten pregnant, I sometimes wonder what would have happened.

The second time I went into VT was during my first half marathon after having given birth to my son Andy. It was the Seaside Half Marathon in Seaside, Florida. I went there for the weekend with Jenn and some other women to relax and race. I was again attempting to train for a half Ironman, and this race was going to be a race to test my fitness in order to see where I was.

It was perfect weather, cool and breezy. Most people were complaining about the temperature, but it was perfect for me. The course was generally pretty flat with a few rolling hills here and there, an easy one for me. When the race started, I went out running at a 7:45 pace. I thought to myself, "Maybe I should slow down. I haven't been in a race in a long time," but I kept going because I felt good, really good. I was able to maintain between a 7:45 and 8:00-minute per mile pace until mile ten, and then something happened.

It was like I hit a brick wall. All of a sudden I felt terrible. My heart rate had been hanging around 150-155 beats per minute (BPM) for most of the run, when suddenly at mile ten it shot up to 220 BPM and then stopped registering altogether on my Garmin watch. I suddenly felt exhausted, anxious, and lightheaded, and my heart was beating out of my chest. I could actually see it beating under my skin.

But I didn't stop. I switched to a walk then a jog until my heart slowed down. I was confused. Again, it never occurred to me something was wrong. As I sit here writing this, I want to yell at myself, "You idiot! Of course there was something wrong! Do you not see the pattern?!" But when you're in the middle of experiencing something, it's never as obvious or as clear as when you look back. There's a reason they say hindsight is twenty-twenty.

Right away, I was disappointed with myself for going out too fast. "I know better! I coach runners!" I kept saying. Then I began questioning the technology. "My heart rate strap must be dirty. My Garmin is broken. Stupid Garmin."

I struggled to finish, but I did. By alternating walking and jogging the last three miles, I finished in 1:52:57. I watched my Garmin the entire time, being sure not to let my heart rate go above 150. I was scared, again.

When I finished, I made excuses about why I hadn't run faster, even though I still had finished ahead of all the women with whom I had come. No one cared that I ran slower than I had planned. The excuses I made weren't for them — they were for me. I never told anyone what had really happened because I was embarrassed.

I was so tired after the race, I had to sleep for a few hours. Again, I should have realized something was up because a half marathon had never been a big deal for me. I usually would be fine getting on a bike afterward and riding an hour or two without an issue. But this time I felt terrible for two days. However, again I thought I had just gone out too fast. The truth is I should have sought medical help that day and didn't. I had a gut feeling something was wrong, but I didn't act on it.

I assumed part of the issue was that I was still breastfeeding, and I attributed being so tired to having a one-year-old. Every time I asked new parents if they were as exhausted as I was, they would all say, "Yes, welcome to parenthood!" However, my severe exhaustion was a warning sign I didn't recognize. I thought it was normal and adjusted my lifestyle so I could get to bed as early 7:30 pm. Another warning sign I ignored was, when I ran fast enough, I experienced heart palpitations, dizziness, and lightheadedness. But it was getting warmer in Atlanta, so I blamed it on the humidity and heat coupled with being a new parent. I had every excuse in the book.

Weeks prior to the Seaside race, there had been a few training runs when I had needed to stop and walk a bit or crouch down in the road to catch my breath. My running partner at the time, Ashley, had recently stopped breastfeeding too and said she felt the same way when she tried to run. She assured me I would feel much better when I finished nursing my son. I couldn't wait to feel good again. I was so tired of feeling sluggish and slow. Everything I was experiencing could be considered normal in isolation or under certain circumstances, such as becoming a new parent. So I kept going and continued to train and race.

A few weeks after the Seaside Half Marathon, I ran the Publix Half Marathon in Atlanta. It would be the last race I would ever run. If I had known it was going to be my last race, I would have gone slower and taken it all in. I would have paid more attention to how each foot felt as it hit the ground. I would have looked into the faces of the crowd as they smiled and cheered. I would have caught the raindrops on my tongue as it poured rather than put a hat on. I wouldn't have felt bad about my time.

I was tired, again. Tired had become the norm for me, so I didn't think much about it. I wanted this race to go better than the previous one, so I decided to ignore my pace and run based only on my heart rate. I was definitely shaken from the last race and needed my confidence back. My intuition said don't push it, and I actually listened this time.

As I ran, I noticed I felt good if I could keep my heart rate around 150 BPM. There were a few times I went above 150 BPM, and I felt a flutter in my chest or a sick feeling in my stomach, so I backed off. I swallowed my pride when I saw a few of my patients pass me on the course, and I stuck to my heart rate rule. I finished faster than my last race and without incident.

I was frustrated that I couldn't run quicker and finish with Ashley, but I had known from the start that wasn't a good idea. Of course, I was still completely exhausted mentally and physically when the race was over. I had to sleep for a few hours after the race, and I never quite got my energy back.

Later that week, when patients and friends asked me how the race had gone, I found myself making excuses for why I had run so slowly. I made the same excuses to myself. Although I was starting to sense that something wasn't right, I still wasn't quite ready to accept there might be something wrong. I was young and otherwise healthy. I had already seen a cardiologist and been given a clean bill of health.

So I continued training for my half Ironman. I swam two to three hours a week, biked four to six hours, and ran four to five days. I had a few days when I didn't feel good, and I had some when I felt great. But my exhaustion was getting worse by the day.

5

The Last Straw

"There is purpose in your season of waiting."

- Megan Smalley

Two years ago today, I had my third episode of ventricular tachycardia. It was my son Andy's first birthday, and I couldn't believe he was already one year old. As I drove Andy to his Montessori school, I thought about the last year and how much our lives had changed.

When I got home, I went out for my five-mile morning run and noticed I was more tired than usual. I had been really tired lately, but today was different. It was worse than usual. I almost didn't go, but I thought I would feel better if I got a few miles under my belt. It was a warm spring morning, and it was just beginning to get humid again. The trees were in full bloom, and the pollen had settled on the sidewalk and cars like a yellow blanket.

I closed my front door, put in my earbuds, and took off running through my neighborhood. I had my favorite Boston Marathon running shorts on and a brand-new pair of shoes. I love the feeling of a new pair of running shoes, and I love the possibility of something great happening when you slide them on for the first time. Not today. Nothing great was about to happen.

During the run, I had to stop several times because I felt "funny." At times it felt like I couldn't breathe. It lasted for a moment, and then it was gone. I would walk a little or crouch down in the road until the feeling passed. I thought it was because I was out of shape so, in typical Kate fashion, I pushed harder. I was annoyed that my body wasn't doing what I wanted it to do. I had been training, had had enough sleep, and wasn't dehydrated.

As the last half-mile of my run approached, I decided to sprint to make up for my less-than-stellar run. As soon as I stopped, it happened. I was standing in front of my house, and I started to get dizzy. I wasn't able to put one foot in front of the other without losing my balance. I felt my heart beating so quickly that it felt like it was beating out of my chest.

I sat down on the front steps of my house, elbows on my knees and head between my elbows. I tried to calm myself down by focusing on my breath. Inhale slowly, exhale slowly, inhale one-two-three, and exhale one-two-three-four. In that moment I thought, "I feel like I am going to die. I better stay outside on my front steps so someone will find me."

My heart was beating so hard and fast that I could see my chest wall moving in and out, in and out rapidly. Looking down, I wondered, "Is that my heart? It can't be!" My heart continued to beat faster and faster. The breathing didn't seem to be helping. My Garmin was having a difficult time registering my heart rate. It flashed numbers that were in the high 200s, 220 then 240, then 250.

After several minutes — I don't really know how long — I got up and started walking toward my neighbor's house. Her front porch wasn't very far away, but I was moving very slowly, trying not to fall down. Then, as I walked up the path and approached her front door, the very rapid heartbeat stopped, and my heart resumed beating normally. I stood outside my neighbor's door for a couple of minutes, making sure the rapid heartbeat didn't come back. I thought, "Maybe this is all in my head. I shouldn't bother Cynthia."

So I turned around and went home. I sat outside for a long time. I was afraid. I knew there was something wrong now, but how serious could it be? After all, I was young, I was an athlete, and I took care of my body. The last time I had seen a cardiologist, they had told me I was fine, that I was just dehydrated. How could anything be wrong?

I called my husband at work and told him what had happened. He asked me if I needed to go to the doctor's. I said I was fine and probably didn't need to go. I downplayed what had happened and told myself I was probably just run down and needed to sleep. I think I called Brian because I wanted someone to tell me to go to the hospital. I don't know why I didn't just go.

I felt so exhausted, but this time I had only gone five miles. I felt anxious for the rest of the day. I would lie down for a little while, and then I would pace around the house for a little while. I went back and forth between lying down and pacing for a few hours.

Then I went to my afternoon Pilates session. I was still feeling "funny" and didn't look like myself. Heather, my instructor and friend, kept asking me if I was okay. Of course I said yes. She didn't really believe me, but I blew it off. I was too afraid to admit that I maybe I wasn't okay.

The next day I went to work and still wasn't feeling well. I got there early, like I always do. I debated saying something to someone, and I eventually asked my colleagues to take my blood pressure. It was low as always, and my heart rate was in the 38-42 range, not an unusually low number for an athlete. Everything seemed fine.

Sitting on a trapeze table in the Pilates area, I explained to my colleagues what had happened on my run. They all looked at me, and I don't think they knew what to do any more than I did. Finally, Julie said, "Cancel your patients and go see your doctor right now." I listened.

I hadn't been to a doctor in so long. I actually don't like to see doctors and had always avoided them at all costs. I had a primary care physician, but when I called, they said I hadn't been there in so long that I couldn't get in. Then I told them I thought I was having an episode of A-fib, so they told me to go to the ER.

I didn't think that was necessary. They were overreacting. So I texted a primary care physician I knew and worked with regularly. He was on vacation and suggested I see his PA. By this time, it was becoming such a pain in the butt to find someone to see that I nearly didn't do anything. However, I was just scared enough that I decided to go to an urgent care facility. I felt so stupid going. I assumed they were going to say I was fine — just under a lot of stress.

Luckily the doctor at Urgent Care recognized something was, in fact, going on and made a few phone calls. He didn't like how low my heart rate was. I knew that wasn't the problem, that my heart rate was always low because of training. However, he was the first doctor to take a second look at me and realize that, even though I was healthy, something was wrong. He got me in to see an electrophysiologist that day. (An electrophysiologist or EP is a cardiologist who specializes in the electric system of the heart.)

I met Dr. Zoubin Alikhani, the EP, that day. When I walked into his office, I was instantly annoyed. The waiting room was packed, and I was the youngest, fittest person there by a long shot. I didn't feel like I belonged there at all. It was obvious how busy the doctor was, but thankfully he squeezed me in.

And, even though he had had to make room in his overbooked schedule to see me, he actually sat down, really listened to what had happened, and talked to me for a long time. He decided I needed some tests, so he asked if I could come back later in the day. Despite not wanting to waste my day in a doctor's office, I did go back and ended up spending the majority of my day in his office. I sat in the maroon leather chairs, pretending to read magazines. I crossed and uncrossed my legs a million times. I checked my email and played on Facebook on my phone. I did everything I could to distract myself from where I was.

I underwent several tests. My echocardiogram looked clear, and I had minor discrepancies on my EKG. Then we did a stress test. When we started the test, I felt fine, and I was passing the test with flying colors, just like I had before. But then Dr. Alikhani saw something and asked me how I felt. I told him I felt fine, but that I could try to make the feeling I had been experiencing on my run happen if he wanted me to.

So I ran on the treadmill and, unlike my previous stress tests, he let me push until I felt what I typically felt on my run. I was running a seven-minute mile on an incline. I made everyone in the room nervous, especially the doctor. He was standing next to me, with one hand pointing at the computer screen and another one stretched out behind me. He even called someone else into the room to stand behind the treadmill just in case.

He was pointing out what he was seeing to his physician's assistant, Leah. As I was running, I was also watching the computer screen. In PT school, we had learned how to read basic EKGs, so I knew enough to know what he was seeing wasn't good. I couldn't believe it was *my* heart I was looking at. I thought, "This isn't real."

That day was the first time any test had shown any irregularities going on with my heart. I am thankful Dr. Alikhani didn't follow the regular stress test protocol that day because otherwise he might not have seen the irregularities. To this day, Zoubin (we're on a first-name basis by now) always brings up how fast I was running on the treadmill and how he had "never seen anything like it," and how he thought I was going to run through the wall.

Even though I saw the EKG as I was running, I was stunned

as I sat in Zoubin's office and he explained to me what was happening. It felt like a bad dream. I only heard parts of what he was saying, even though I tried very hard to listen to every word. At the time, he didn't have a specific diagnosis. He simply told me that my heart was going into idiopathic (this is the medical field's way of saying they have no idea what is causing something) ventricular tachycardia, and we had to find out why.

He strongly urged me to be careful and to stop running. I was furious. I didn't want to stop running or exercising. He told me he thought marathon running was crazy, and that made me even angrier. I now know he did the right thing, but I wasn't in a place I could hear it back then. He wanted to run more tests and figure out why I was having VT, and he needed more data to put the full picture together.

We ended up compromising that day in his office. He said I could keep exercising, but I had to keep my heart rate under 150 BPM at all times. And he wanted me to exercise in a group or with a friend instead of alone. I was so angry with him. It wasn't his fault, but he was the only other person in the room, and I was scared. I was also frustrated. I told him that I was training for a half Ironman and fully intended to compete. Once again, my stubbornness and pure defiance were not my best traits that day, but I used them to protect myself. Zoubin handled me well and, even though he didn't understand me, he listened.

I left his office defeated. I was exhausted, anxious, and scared. My husband was out of town on business, so I called him and told him that I would be having more tests and that something was wrong. Brian was concerned and asked if he needed to come home, but I told him not to worry about it. None of it seemed real.

I called Jenn and Scott instead, and they came over and took care of me. Scott picked Andy up from school, and Jenn sat with me on the couch while I cried. I felt numb and wanted to wake up from the nightmare I was experiencing. I had a hard time falling asleep that night and every night afterward for months.

The following day, I got up and went to work. I let my colleagues know that something was wrong, but I wasn't sure what it was. All I wanted to do was go for a long, hard run to blow off steam, but I was afraid to. So I didn't do any running or other exercise for at least a week.

It's terrible to know that something serious is wrong with you, but you have no idea what it is. From March to August of that year was the most difficult time for me. I suffered from a lot of anxiety, exhaustion, and sleep deprivation. I was worried and afraid I could die at any moment. I didn't ever want to be alone. Whenever my husband was out of town traveling, it was exponentially worse. I would lie awake at night with all the lights on, afraid to fall asleep. I was afraid I would die in my sleep, and my son would be alone, crying in his crib, and no one would find him.

I went through test after test with no answers. I was exhausted. I hated going to the doctor's office, but I was there all the time. I stopped seeing friends and answering calls or even text messages. I didn't want to try to explain what was going on with me. I didn't want to make plans anymore. I wanted to be left alone.

As March turned into April and then May, I would drive to work and sit in my car outside the office, but I couldn't go in. I tried. I could see people through the windows working and hoped they didn't see me. I didn't want to miss another day or cancel another patient, but I couldn't do it. I couldn't go in. I would call the front office from the car, have them cancel my patients, and then drive home, get in my pajamas, and sleep all day.

I'm not sure why working was so difficult for me. Maybe it was because I was treating runners and triathletes all day long. I couldn't bear the idea of giving it all up or having to explain to someone why I wasn't racing or why my half Ironman training had come to a halt. Maybe it was the stress that I put on myself to do everything at 150 percent, and I was afraid I wouldn't be able to deliver that kind of effort to my work. Or maybe it was the competitive, high-stress environment I was working in. One of the core values of our office was excellence, but in our office excellence meant perfection, and perfection is exhausting. It didn't matter why I couldn't go in. The fact was I couldn't go in. I just couldn't.

When I was able to go to work, it was difficult. People were concerned but didn't know how to talk to me about it. I felt like everyone was walking on eggshells around me or giving me the "you poor thing" look. Patients would ask me when my next race was, and I would feel guilty for not running. Sometimes I would explain what was going on, and I would hear things like, "They will figure this out, and you will be fine," or "Don't worry, you'll be running races in no time."

Deep down I knew I wouldn't be, but I didn't have the

heart to tell them (or myself) or the energy to go into it any further. I just smiled and nodded my head. I think they were thankful. They didn't want to pursue it any further either.

I had started to run a little bit again and was happy to at least be outside. I ran slowly and kept my heart rate under 140 BPM just to give me a little buffer from the lower-than-150 BPM Zoubin had advised I could do. I was nervous enough that, for once in my life, I didn't want to push it.

There were many nights I found myself waking up in the middle of the night, and I wouldn't be able to fall back to sleep. I would be up for hours, trying so hard to sleep, but I couldn't. I would lie there, staring into the darkness, willing myself to just try to get one more hour of sleep. I would get up and pace around our dining room downstairs or try to read a book or do something, anything, to distract myself. The next morning, my husband would wake up rested, and I would feel like hell. I tried not to take it out on him, but I would get so angry that he could sleep and I couldn't. There is no doubt that all those sleepless nights added to my overall fatigue and anxiety.

It wasn't just at night that I felt bad. I would feel my heart palpitating just sitting on the couch. It was horrible. I would get my Garmin out to see if I was freaking out for no reason or if my heart really was all over the place. And, of course, the more I paid attention to my heart rate, the worse it got.

Even though Zoubin said I could call him anytime, I didn't want to bother him, so I didn't. I felt like I was overreacting and that this wasn't really happening. I was convinced he had so many people much worse off to manage. I was in serious denial.

Memorial Day weekend, my husband was away for a

bachelor party. He wasn't sure if he should go, but I encouraged him to. I told him not to worry, that I'd be just fine. It was hot and humid all weekend. Saturday, I went for a slow five- to six-mile run, swam in the pool for about forty-five minutes, and did a lot of walking with my son. I followed the rules Zoubin had set. I kept my heart rate between 140-150 BPM and "took it easy." A five-mile run and a forty-five-minute swim followed by two hours of walking was taking it easy for me. I remember being tired in the pool and thinking I needed a nap.

Prior to leaving for his trip, Brian had arranged for his parents to take Andy for one night to give me a little break. Feeling tired, I drove Andy over to his grandparents, kissed him goodbye, and went home. That evening, I met a friend downtown for music and wine on the square. We put a blanket out on the grass, caught up, and had a couple glasses of red wine. Then I walked home and went to bed. I wasn't even tipsy.

I had a hard time falling asleep because I was completely alone. I left the light on in my room and finally dozed off. Then, a few hours later, I woke up. My heart was racing, and I could feel fluttering in my chest. I felt strange and started questioning whether I was having chest and arm pain or not. I paced around my room for a little while and then got up and went downstairs.

I debated for several minutes if I should bother anyone. Eventually, I sent a few text messages, but no one responded, probably because it was one in the morning. I started to freak out just enough, so I finally called my friends Ashley and Philip. Ashley works in the cardiac ICU at Children's Hospital, so I think I assumed she was going to tell me I was fine. Instead, she suggested I go to the ER.

She had to go to work in a few hours, and their daughter was sound asleep. So a few minutes later, Philip pulled up in front of my house in his truck and took me to the closest ER. I apologized profusely because I was so embarrassed. I thought I was probably overreacting and wondered if I should have driven myself. I felt so pathetic for having to wake people up in the middle of the night. I didn't feel good, but I didn't actually think anything was wrong.

Philip and I sat in the ER for a long time. It wasn't a pleasant place. I didn't like the smell, the bathrooms were disgusting, and I looked around, thinking, "I don't belong here. I'm fine." I even wondered several times if we should leave. Then they finally called my name.

After a few blood tests, an EKG, and a lot of waiting, I was thankful to have a friend with me, but I was still embarrassed. Finally, the results came back. I tested positive for elevated troponin in my blood, which indicates a possible heart attack, and I was admitted to the hospital.

Up until that point, I hadn't called my husband. I didn't want to bother Brian while he was away with his friends, and, besides, I thought it was probably nothing. In fact, I had almost convinced myself that the whole trip to the ER was one big mistake. However, after I was admitted, Philip tried to persuade me several times to call Brian. Finally I did, albeit grudgingly.

Brian answered his phone, and I explained what had happened. Without hesitation, he jumped in the car in Texas, drove a few hours to the nearest airport, and got on the next flight home to Atlanta, making it back within twelve hours of when I called him. In the meantime, Philip stayed with me for several hours until I told him I was really okay, and then he went home.

In the hospital, they gave me a beta blocker, and it was so strong that I could barely get out of bed. I tried to tell the nurses and the doctor I didn't want a beta blocker, but I was too out of it to protest. My heart rate was already very low from my being an endurance athlete, but then the medicine decreased it even more, making it difficult for me to function or even get out of bed. I felt like I was in and out of consciousness, but I wasn't sure if it was the medicine, my heart, or that I was completely exhausted. My blood pressure, also normally very low, got low enough that my monitors were constantly beeping. The nurses came in and out, turning the monitors off, but sometimes the beeping would go on forever. Finally, I started turning it off myself. I knew how to do it from the acute care rotations I had done while in PT school.

The next morning, when Jenn and Scott, our good friends and Andy's godparents, found out I was in the hospital, they came right over and took good care of me. Jenn didn't leave my side. I think it was she who finally said something about the beta blocker being too strong because I was so out of it. When I was awake, we lay in bed watching Netflix episodes of *The Mindy Project*, trying to take our minds off what was actually happening.

Hours later, after they stopped giving me the beta blocker, I walked up and down the hall over and over again, almost daring them to tell me to rest. I didn't like being in the hospital and felt like a prisoner. I wanted to leave and for them to tell me I was fine.

I never minded being in hospitals when I was working in them, but being on the other side was more than difficult, and I didn't feel like I belonged there. The hospital wasn't restful. The bed was uncomfortable, and the room was always too hot or too cold. Every time I fell asleep, I was woken up to have my vitals checked or to make sure I was okay. The food was terrible. It was unhealthy and tasted like cafeteria food from high school.

Zoubin was out of town on vacation, so another doctor from his group took care of me. No matter what questions I asked, no one seemed to know what to tell me. I was a mess. I could no longer ignore that something was seriously wrong.

I ended up spending two nights in the hospital and went through more testing. They decided to do a nuclear stress test on me, which was much worse than any of the tests I had previously experienced. For this procedure, they had to take me downstairs in a wheelchair, even though I protested and wanted to walk. Then I sat in the drab hallway of the hospital basement in a line of people, all older than me, all in wheelchairs and waiting for the test to be done. The longer I waited, the more frustrated and agitated I got.

Finally, when it was my turn, they wheeled me into a dimly lit room where there was a technician, a doctor, some computers, and a hospital bed. I was told to get into the hospital bed so they could administer the test. Then they proceeded to inject me with a drug that caused my heart rate to increase rapidly. It was terrible. I felt like I was trying to catch my breath but couldn't. My heart began to race, and I couldn't control what was happening. The test was short but uncomfortable.

Afterward, they rolled me back into the hall, and I had to

wait for someone to take me back to my room. A few hours later, the doctor came in to tell me that they hadn't found anything and that he still couldn't give me any answers, so I was being discharged.

A week later, I went back to work. I was more uneasy than previously because not only did no one know what was wrong with me, but I wasn't getting better. In fact, I was getting worse. The following week, on Friday, I felt terrible again, my pulse was thready, and I could feel the fluttering in my chest. I asked my colleague and friend Julie to feel my pulse and take a look at me. She told me to cancel my last patient and call Zoubin. I was so sick of being sick!

I called him and went to his office. In typical Atlanta fashion, there was a traffic issue. A small plane had landed on the highway and had blocked traffic on Route 285, one of the major highways around Atlanta. The traffic was so bad that I couldn't get to Zoubin's office, so he had me see his colleague at another office. His colleague gave me fluids, talked to me for a while, and decided I might have something called POTS (Postural Orthostatic Tachycardia Syndrome). He changed my medication and told me to drink an unbelievable amount of water, eat a lot of sodium, and see how I did.

I left the office feeling a bit confused and surprised. I had never heard of POTS, but he was a cardiologist, so I thought maybe he was right. And at least it was an answer! I didn't have any salt in my house, so I had to buy it. For several weeks, I drank excessive amounts of fluids and ate excessive amounts of salt. I drank pickle juice before I swam or ran as instructed. My fingers became so swollen they felt like sausages, and the next time I went to the doctor's office I had gained nearly five pounds!

In the back of my mind, I knew I didn't have POTS, but I convinced myself maybe I did because at least it was a diagnosis. When I went back to see Zoubin, he confirmed my suspicion that I didn't have POTS and took me off the medication. I was glad I could stop eating salt, but I continued to be frustrated because we still didn't have any answers.

I was so frustrated that I didn't know where to turn, so I decided to go see an integrative medicine doctor. An integrative medicine doctor is a holistic physician who combines typical western medical treatment with holistic medicine, herbs, and supplements. I thought, "Why not? It can't hurt." Perhaps she would discover something different that could help me.

When I went to see Dr. Grossman, I was beyond exhausted. I was no longer able to sleep through the night, and my brain wouldn't turn off. I had dark circles around my eyes from lack of sleep. Every chance I got, I would lie down and rest. I wasn't talking to my friends anymore, and I felt quite isolated. At this point, I had given up drinking caffeine, was staying away from chocolate because of the caffeine and red wine (it can give you something called premature ventricular contractions or PVCs), and barely running or exercising anymore. Everything I loved was slowly being taken away. I was at my wit's end.

The integrative medicine office was pleasantly different from any other doctor's office I had been to. When I first walked in, someone greeted me and offered me some tea. Then I sat in a nice comfy chair and, instead of annoying advertisements playing on a television, there was quiet, meditative music playing in the background. It was the first doctor's appointment I had been to in months when I wasn't angry. Maybe it was the atmosphere or maybe I was just too exhausted to fight anymore.

Dr. Grossman came in and took an extensive medical history. She was very nice and very thorough, but she too seemed baffled at what had been going on with me. I had several panels of blood work done to test for adrenal fatigue, hormones, allergies — you name it, I had it tested that day! The doctor gave me some supplements and advised me to stop doing work after dinner and to start drinking tart cherry juice at night before bed to improve my sleep hygiene.

On the way home from the appointment, I stopped at a health food store to pick up some dandelion tea and other supplements she had suggested. I hadn't eaten, so I ate some food from the hot bar. When I got home, I made the tea, and within twenty minutes I was throwing up. After throwing up a few times, I had to go pick my son up from school. As we were getting close to home, I started to feel sick again. I ran through the front door, leaving it wide open, holding Andy on one hip while holding my hair with the other, and I began throwing up into the toilet.

Luckily Brian came home early and found me holding a crying toddler as I threw up. He took Andy, and I spent the next few hours lying on the bathroom floor and then trying to crawl into the guest bedroom nearby. At first, I thought it was the tea that had made me sick. Then I thought perhaps it was the supplements I had taken. But then I realized I must have gotten food poisoning from the hot bar at the health food store, of all places! For nearly twenty-four hours, I felt like a truck had hit me. All I could think was, "REALLY?! What else can possibly go wrong?!"

I ended up seeing Dr. Grossman twice. Her suggestions did help with my sleep hygiene, and I did have a little more energy, but, ultimately, she didn't have any answers either. I continued to feel more hopeless but didn't want to give up. I continued to search for answers anywhere I could find them.

In addition to my general practitioner, Zoubin, and Dr. Grossman, I eventually got another appointment with a sports cardiologist, Dr. Jonathan Kim. He was suggested to me by a friend with whom I had worked in the medical tent for the Peachtree Road Race. Dr. Kim was highly recommended as someone to see if you were an athlete. I wanted to consult with a physician who understood athletes and how important exercise was to me. I was excited to see him because I thought, "He will understand. He will let me run and tell me nothing is wrong!"

I liked Jonathan right away, but he didn't know what was going on either. I went through another battery of tests, this time with both my cardiologists working together. I had more EKGs and ended up having two MRIs; another echocardiogram; a stress test; exercise testing; wore a Holter monitor for twenty-four hours, forty-eight hours, and then a month; and probably had more testing I don't remember now. If you have ever been through multiple medical tests, you know what it's like. Appointments suck up all your free time, people are poking and prodding you at every moment, and you feel less and less like yourself.

Holter monitors are very intrusive, but they are a great tool for collecting data about your heart, so cardiologists love them. You are set up with the monitor in the office, and you have to wear the same sticky pads with wires attached that you wear for an EKG, only you're wearing them all day and all night. When you're sleeping, you have to find a place to put the little monitor so you don't get tangled in the wires or pull off a pad. When you wear a twenty-four- or forty-eight-hour monitor you aren't allowed to shower. If it's warm outside and you want to wear a tank top, everyone can see the wiring sticking out and the box on your hip. When you're wearing a Holter monitor, you can't pretend you are fine anymore. People stare, look away, or ask questions. I hated wearing it.

The results of all my testing revealed nothing obvious, so we kept looking. In the meantime, I kept feeling terrible. I was so tired. I don't think exhaustion is a strong enough word to describe how much fatigue I was experiencing. Every time I felt my heart beat or flutter, I would hold my breath and be terrified something bad was about to happen. I convinced myself I could die at any moment, and then my son would grow up and wouldn't even remember me. I tried so hard to put on a good face, to keep going to work every day and seeing patients, to be a good mother and a good wife. Some days, it was all I could do to get out of bed. I cried a lot.

I needed help. Not just medical help but psychological help. I had always thought asking for help was a weakness, but I knew I couldn't keep going on as I was. While all my health issues were unfolding, my friend Julie was also having medical challenges, and I noticed how well she seemed to be handling it. She told me she had been talking with a life coach and that it was helping her a lot.

Julie told me she too had been having difficulties with anxiety, stress, and sleep, and her life coach had suggested she start adding a few drops of valerian root to her water before bed. I tried it and was finally able to sleep a little with less frequent episodes of waking up in a panic. I started to think that maybe there was something to having a life coach. I eventually got up the courage to email Julie's coach and ask for help. It was one of the best decisions I ever made.

6

Diagnosis

"I spent a lot of years trying to outrun or outsmart vulnerability by making things certain and definite, black and white, good and bad...[this] limited the fullness of those important experiences that are wrought with uncertainty: Love, belonging, trust, joy, and creativity to name a few."

- Brené Brown

The first day I spoke to my life coach, Dr. Shawn Haywood, was the day after I had been throwing up for hours and lying on my cold bathroom floor with food poisoning. I was exhausted, my head hurt, and I was at an ultimate low point. I still had no idea what was wrong with me, and I knew the road ahead was going to be full of more obstacles. I was slightly skeptical that the coach would be able to help me, but I was hopeful at the same time.

Shawn's and my first conversation was to make sure we would be compatible. It was nothing like I expected. I called her from my guest room floor, propped up against the linen bench at the end of the bed. No one else was home, but for some reason I felt like I had to hide. It was probably a deep-rooted fear of failure — of finally having to ask for help. Despite my reservations, I was comfortable with Shawn immediately and quickly realized how good it felt to just talk to someone.

I had spent my whole life trying to keep people at arm's length so as not to hurt, not to feel too much, in order to be the best at everything I did, to win, to do the right thing, to be . . . perfect. I no longer had the energy to live this way, and Shawn met me exactly where I was. As I hung up the phone that night, I let out a sigh. I had been holding my breath for so long, and I hadn't even known it.

Over time, Shawn has helped me with so many things. She helped me gain perspective and find some goodness in what I was going through. She made me realize that your life is the sum of your choices. You can choose to be stressed out all the time, to continue to be a part of a job or a relationship that you do not love, to beat yourself up over every little thing OR you can choose to be happy, grateful, authentic, stress-free (or close to it), and live in the present.

Now, don't get the wrong idea. This process of teaching myself how to think and how to live in a different way isn't easy. My work has just begun. So far, Shawn has been and continues to be a steady voice and a safe place as everything around me has been challenged and changed.

She gave me a metaphorical mirror, and I was able to

reflect on what was happening. I quickly realized that I was surrounded by so much unnecessary stress. I loved my job, but the culture was rooted in perfectionism. Going to work was stressful. I felt like I had to give 150 percent all the time with no end in sight. Also, we were paid based on collections, so there was too much competition and not enough compassion and collaboration among colleagues. Then at home, I would beat myself up if I was even a few minutes late picking up Andy from school or if I couldn't make it to every event. I would think I was a bad mom if I didn't stop everything and play with him every second. I didn't even want to cook dinner if it meant he was playing by himself.

I started to recognize the unhealthy habits I had created around perfectionism and fear. I had unrealistic expectations of myself, and then, when I couldn't meet those expectations, I would think I wasn't good enough. I would tell myself I had to complete all nine hundred tasks on my to-do list and then go to bed late, wake up early, and, as a result, not take care of myself.

I recognized that I needed to start prioritizing my health, my family, and myself. The only way I could do this was to start letting go. I had to learn that the world wouldn't end if my to-do list didn't get finished. That sleep was more important and allowed me to function better the next day. I had to tell myself that it wasn't realistic to put 150 percent into everything I did because then I would end up depleted, with nothing left for my family or myself. I had to decide what was really important to me and let go of the things that were no longer helpful.

I learned that sometimes the dishes won't get done and the laundry may not be folded, but it's okay. One of my homework assignments from Shawn was to throw away 80 percent of all the academic journals I kept (there were piles everywhere) just in case I wanted to read them again and again. These changes were all very difficult for me to accept. The more I saw how I was living, the more I knew this meant more change was coming, whether I liked it or not.

It took nine months to diagnose what was wrong with me. While my doctors were trying to put together the pieces of my medical condition, I felt like I was slowly losing pieces of myself each day, week, and month that passed without any answers. At least I was still allowed to exercise. It wasn't what I considered much exercise, but it was better than nothing. The doctors didn't want to take everything away from me, but they wanted to keep me safe. So I had a lot of rules.

I continued to run, bike, and swim. I was running with my heart rate at less than 130 BPM (an eleven- or twelve-minute mile), walking up hills, and going on runs that were only three to four miles long. I was used to running seven- to eight-minute miles, sprinting up hills, and going on runs that lasted for hours. I was frustrated! So frustrated that sometimes I wanted to scream and stomp my feet. I wanted to be so loud that everyone around me would hear and feel my frustration. But I didn't say a word. I held my feelings in, which didn't help, but I didn't know that yet.

On the one hand, I was embarrassed that I wasn't out there killing it all the time. On the other hand, every time I went for a run, I wondered if I'd make it home. My runs became less enjoyable, and I became more fearful that I was going to go into tachycardia.

When friends or patients asked me how I felt, I hated telling them the truth. So I often told them what they wanted to hear and what I wanted to be true. "I feel good." And they always responded, "Don't worry. You'll get back out there in no time." I didn't want to admit that I knew it was a very real possibility I would never get back out there the way I used to.

One day, I was about a mile in on a run, when I felt it. I felt that all-too-familiar feeling of my heart skipping a beat, and then I couldn't catch my breath. It wasn't a strong sensation, and my heart wasn't beating fast, but it was there. I had been running slowly, only ten- to eleven-minute miles, so I couldn't believe it. Tears started to well up in my eyes, and, before I knew it, they were streaming down my face and into my mouth. I tried to wipe them away quickly before anyone noticed, even though I was alone. No one was there to see my tears, and no one was there to understand my tears. I stopped running and walked the rest of the route, feeling utterly defeated. I didn't run much after that.

I swam every Wednesday at noon with the Atlanta Triathlon Club. I had built my work schedule around my workouts so that every week I could leave the office and swim at Mercer University with the group. I hadn't been a member of the club very long before I started having problems, so I didn't feel very comfortable telling anyone what was going on with me. If I missed a few days, a few people would ask where I had been, but normally no one seemed to notice. The coach tried to have me move into a faster lane on more than one occasion, but I told him I couldn't and stayed with the beginner swimmers. I was worried that something would happen at a faster pace, and

I felt safer with the slower, less-advanced group.

By this time, my outdoor bike rides had stopped altogether. I would get on my indoor trainer one or two times a week, but it wasn't the same as riding with a group or riding to meet a goal or train for a race. I tried to enjoy myself, but it was difficult.

The same rule about my heart rate applied to riding as it did to running. I had to keep it below 130 BPM. This was much easier on the bike, and I felt safer because I rode at home when someone was usually there. Some days I took my trainer out back onto the stone patio, faced it toward the green grass and flowers in the backyard, and rode outside just to be able to enjoy the sun and breeze. I could at least smile and forget a little on those days.

If Brian was out of town or at work, I would call or walk over to my neighbor Cynthia's house or call Jenn to let someone know I was exercising and to check on me later. However, despite my desire to keep exercising, I was losing steam. It wasn't as much fun when I had so many limitations, and I was really scared something would happen. It felt like I was trying to hold on to something, but I didn't even know anymore what it was I was holding on to.

Running, and especially running marathons, had become an escape for me a long time ago. It had helped me get through my childhood, and it had helped me find myself when I was all but lost. It had been a way to calm my mind, dispel my nervousness, and control my life. And I had loved running as any good type A personality would.

Losing my ability to run was weighing heavily on me. Not only did I struggle with all of the health challenges, but day by day I was losing both my coping mechanism and myself. Several months into my journey, and before I knew my diagnosis, Shawn asked me if I still needed to exercise like I used to.

We had been working together a lot, and I had already made many positive changes in my life. I had thrown away all those old academic journals, and after reading a new one, I threw it away too. I set timers while working at home that made me stop before eight or nine at night so I could get sleep or spend more time with Brian. I even told myself things like, "I get to fold the laundry," instead of, "I have to fold the laundry."

When Shawn asked me if I needed to exercise, I immediately thought, "Of course I still need to exercise! Are you crazy?! Who doesn't need this much exercise? How could I possibly give it up completely?"

Hours after we hung up, I was still thinking about what she had said, and it was beginning to resonate with me. She had said, "If you create stillness on the inside, recognize the madness in your mind that keeps saying it's not enough, and then let it go, you may find you don't need to exercise the way you used to." She had gone on to challenge me to ask myself what all this nervousness was about and then to, "Embrace the feelings that are coming, revealing more of your authenticity and shedding the layers of your grief." She pointed out that I kept physically pushing myself over the edge rather than dealing with my emotions.

And that's when I learned how to cry again. I realized that instead of letting my emotions flow, I had always run away from them as fast as I could. I had run away from fear, anxiety, nervousness, change, and pain my entire life rather than facing them. By not facing my feelings each time they arose, they intensified, and I had to run faster and farther to get away from them.

However, on the flip side, running had also been my platform to clear my head, decompress, imagine great ideas, and make unbelievable friendships. It had taught me that I could do whatever I set out to do and that even I had a breaking point. Losing running and endurance sports was helping me face the very things that had driven me to compete and push harder. But I still had to grieve my loss.

I am what Shawn might refer to as a recovering perfectionist. My entire life, every time I was faced with a challenge I was able to get through it and move forward. But I was never satisfied with my performance until it was perfect or looked perfect to everyone else around me. The more out of control I felt, the more important it was for me to have things and people around me be perfect. I was the type of person who cleaned before the cleaners came and straightened the pictures on the wall after they left. There was even a time when my closet was perfectly organized by color and length of sleeve. Shawn has helped me realize that there is no perfect. No matter what I do, it doesn't exist, and it never will.

Perfect is an illusion. As author Brené Brown states, "Perfectionism is a 20-ton shield that we carry around." Nothing gets in and nothing gets out. Perfectionism has caused me so much unnecessary stress, self-doubt, pain, and suffering. I was running through life as fast as I could, holding up my 20-ton shield in front of me to block all the hurt, fear, anxiety, and shame, but also all the joy and happiness. When I no longer had the energy to hold up my shield and I no longer had the ability to run, I nearly crumpled.

In July, I had an endocardial VT ablation. This is an outpatient procedure performed by an electrophysiologist to destroy tissue in the heart that's allowing incorrect electrical signals that lead to abnormal heart rhythms. Prior to the procedure, I was excited because I thought it would fix the problem, and I would be able to get back to my life. But I was also nervous because Zoubin was going to burn part of my heart. Prior to the surgery, Shawn asked me to consider that it might not fix everything. I didn't want to consider that option at all, but she had planted a seed and had tried to prepare me.

The night before the procedure, Andy slept over at his grandparents' house. I kissed and snuggled him as long as I could before Brian and I had to go home. Then we tried to fall asleep, but for a long time we just lay there, holding each other and staring into each other's eyes. We were both hopeful and frightened.

The next morning, we woke up early and headed to St. Joseph's Hospital in Atlanta. After we had completed all the paperwork, I went back into the pre-op area for patients undergoing procedures. I put my clothes and belongings in a clear plastic bag with the hospital's name on it and got dressed in a hospital gown and blue surgical cap. The nurses prepared the surgical site in my groin, near the femoral artery. I was hooked up to an EKG machine, a blood pressure cuff, and I had an oximeter on my finger to monitor my heart rate and oxygen. The monitors kept sounding an alarm because my heart rate was so low. I couldn't see very well because I had taken out my contacts since I would be under anesthesia for several hours. I was nervous, but so hopeful that this would be the end of all the stress and confusion.

Zoubin came in to tell me that everything looked good and we would be done in no time. He was empathetic and looked hopeful. As I lay in the hospital bed, they wheeled me back to the hearth catheterization lab. The room was a typical sterile operating room, and it was cold. To my left, there was a white board with my name, age, and procedure type written on it. Next to my name, someone had drawn a stick figure of a woman running. It made me smile. Everyone seemed very nice.

They put pads on my chest and back, hooked me up to monitors, and there was a lot of small talk as they tried to make me feel better. Eventually I lay down on the operating table, and they put me into twilight sleep. I was in and out. I could hear the monitor, and I could intermittently see or hear the people around me.

Then they had to take me slightly out of the twilight sleep in order to induce VT. I felt cold and anxious while my heart would beat very fast and then calm down. My body began to shake uncontrollably. I tried to think about this experience the way I would think about racing. If I could just get through it, I'd be fine.

I had no idea how long I was in there, and I was glad when it was all over. They wheeled me back to the recovery area, and I slowly started to come to. My leg was sore from where the catheter had entered my femoral artery, and I was a little wobbly, but overall okay.

Brian came back to see me. He had been in the waiting

room for several hours together with his parents. He had a look of relief on his face, but something was weighing on him. Zoubin had apparently already talked to them while I was recovering and before he came to check on me. Zoubin told me what he had told Brian, that he had done as much as he could, but he hadn't been able to get everything. My VT was more complicated because the node that was misfiring was located in a spot that was very difficult and possibly too risky to get to. I was discouraged immediately. I knew this meant there was a possibility that undergoing the procedure wouldn't solve all my problems.

I went home that night, and Andy stayed with his grandparents for a few days so I could recover. Brian and I took it easy. I was tired, and my leg was sore. But four days later, Andy was home, and we still had our traditional Tour de France party at our home. I didn't do as much and spent more time on the couch than usual, but the party was still a lot of fun.

Over the next few weeks, I began to notice I felt significantly better. My exhaustion was minimal, and Brian even said things like, "There you are! I missed my wife!" I was able to play with Andy and go to work without having to go to bed at 7:30. I was so happy. I even allowed myself to start dreaming about running and training again. I started looking into half and full Ironman races scheduled for the following year. After about a week, I went out for a few short and easy runs, and they felt okay. I was beginning to think the nightmare was over.

Several weeks later, I saw Jonathan, my sports cardiologist, for a follow-up exercise stress test. I couldn't wait to go because I thought I'd be given the green light to slowly return to my old life. I got on the treadmill and started jogging. I didn't feel great, but I hadn't been running very much. Then Jonathan asked if I was okay. I said I felt something but was fine. He stopped the test.

I was still on a very low dose of flecainide, an anti-arrhythmic medication, but I was going into VT on the treadmill. It wasn't obvious to me, but the feeling was similar to how I felt when I would crouch down during a run or before I would pass out. I wasn't given the okay to return to full exercise. I was told to keep my heart rate low while I was running and to take it easy.

Several weeks later, I went in for my second ablation procedure. Zoubin warned me that it might not work, but in my mind that was not an option. Of course it was going to work. It had to work! Brian's parents took care of Andy again, and I planned for a few days off from work.

When I got to the hospital, all the nurses recognized me and greeted me warmly, asking me what I was doing back there. It was strangely comforting that they recognized me and were so kind. Since the procedure was the same as the last one, I was hooked up to the same monitors. This time I played a game with myself. How low could I get my heart rate to go by focusing on my breathing and how often could I make the monitors beep. It was a fun way for me to pass the time. Then one of the nurses came in to print out the EKG. She looked a little surprised. Then Leah, Zoubin's PA, came in and looked at it. They tried not to make me nervous, but it was too late. I knew something was up.

Zoubin came in and looked at the data, and I could tell he

was debating what to do. He said that my EKG looked different than the last time, and he wasn't sure about the ablation. I could feel the tears welling up in my eyes and tried not to cry. I was able to hold them back and shook my head. Finally, he decided to take me back to the Cath Lab to see what he could do.

When I got there, they prepped me like before, but something was different. Zoubin came in and told me he would like to give me adrenaline to see what my heart did before he attempted the procedure. He was in a room watching the monitors, and I started to notice other physicians and people gathering in the room. I couldn't really see them, but I could hear their voices whispering.

Getting adrenaline pumped into your system is like drinking ten Starbucks coffees at once. Your heart is racing, your palms get sweaty, and it is incredibly uncomfortable. But I didn't care if it meant he could do the procedure. I held on for as long as I could, just hoping the surgery would take place. It didn't.

Once they saw my EKG on adrenaline, they stopped everything and brought me back to the recovery room. I was heartbroken because I knew this meant something was truly wrong with me. I wasn't going to go back to my life as I had known it before. I think that's when I started to feel depressed. I was thankful to have Shawn and Brian for support, but it was hard for me to verbalize even to them how I felt.

We were back to the drawing board. My doctors were now reconsidering things they had previously ruled out. I had more tests, including a genetic test. Once I had a test, it would take several weeks or sometimes even a few months to get the results.

My friend Corey, who is a massage therapist, had mentioned a few times that she might be looking for someone with whom to share space. Each time she said something, I heard her but never imagined opening my own physical therapy practice. It felt too scary and unpredictable. When I told Shawn about it, she encouraged me to pursue it. Initially, I laughed at her and thought she was insane.

However, there were days I drove to work and couldn't go in. Days I was so anxious all I could do was cry. Nights I woke up every hour, afraid I was going to die in the middle of the night. I couldn't keep living like this. I knew I needed to do something, to create something, and to have space to just be. If I couldn't put my energy into running and triathlon, I needed another outlet.

When I first mentioned having my own PT practice to Brian, he nearly lost it. I can still remember where we were when I told him and the look on his face. It was the beginning of fall, and there were leaves on the ground. I was sitting in one of the black metal chairs in our backyard, playing with Andy and throwing a ball to our dog Austin. Brian had just gotten home from work and was exhausted from his commute. Before I even knew what I was saying, I blurted out, "I think I might quit my job. Shawn thinks I should open my own practice."

At first, he said nothing. Then he started pacing at the top of the stairs on our porch. I knew he wanted to say what he was thinking, but he was trying so hard to be supportive. It was very clear he thought I was losing my mind. He even said something like, "Are you sure Shawn knows what she's talking about? Maybe you shouldn't be talking to her so much."

Several weeks later, I had decided it was the right thing to do. Brian and I talked it out, mapped it out, and decided we could try it and see what happened. Once he heard me out and realized it might actually work, Brian agreed. Once he agreed, I decided it might actually be a bad idea. In the end, it was Brian who encouraged me to move forward with it. We were both nervous.

A few days later, while face down on Corey's massage table, I asked, "Are you serious about sharing your space?" Luckily she was, and over the next few months we worked out some of the details. One day in October, I gave notice. Leaving my job was difficult because I loved the people I worked with. I had always thought I'd work there for years and years. But I knew I had to quit for my mental and physical health, and so I did.

I opened my own practice, Precision Performance and Physical Therapy, located in The Center for Love and Light. At the time, I had no idea what a profound effect this would have on me. My intention was to see a few people — just enough so I could pay the bills, and that was it. I was so burned out and exhausted that I felt like I needed to hide.

Once again, Shawn pushed me to think bigger than that, and I laughed at her, telling her she was insane. I was never going to have enough patients to do more than pay my bills. The intention was to continue working, but build a space where I could manage my stress, anxiety, and workload. I imagined opening my own practice as a project to make me happy. I would be able to continue doing what I loved, on my own terms, in an environment filled with love, calm, and support.

Then I got a call from Jonathan, the sports cardiologist, a

week before I was due to leave my old job. He had gotten the results back from the genetic testing, wanted me to come into the office, and asked if Brian could come with me. The rest of this memory isn't completely clear. However, I will share it even though it may not be exactly the way it happened.

When Jonathan called, I knew it wasn't good news. I had become very close to both Zoubin and Jonathan over the past several months and knew them well. They had been so supportive and empathetic, and I felt like they truly cared about what happened to me. Because of our relationship, I asked Jonathan to just tell me the truth. I could handle it. He didn't want to, but he did anyway. He said he wanted us to come into the office as soon as we could, but my genetic testing had come back positive, and I was officially diagnosed with arrhythmogenic right ventricular cardiomyopathy (ARVC).

I was quiet on the phone and probably in a bit of shock. I hung up and just sat where I was for a long time. Then I got up and went about my day.

ARVC is a very rare, progressive, genetic heart disease. It is a disease of the cardiac muscle and primarily affects the right ventricle but can occasionally affect both. Over time, cardiac cells break and die, leaving scar tissue to form on the outside of the ventricle. These scars can cause arrhythmia (abnormal timing or rhythm of the heartbeat). Also, as the disease progresses and more scars form, the heart begins having a difficult time pumping. Severity and progression of the disease varies but can ultimately lead to heart transplant or death.

According to Johns Hopkins, the leader in ARVC research, the disease accounts for up to one-fifth of sudden cardiac deaths in people less than thirty-five years of age. It is more prevalent in the athletic population. If you carry the gene, the more hours you have spent exercising, the higher risk you have for developing the disease. ARVC is not only rare but also difficult to diagnose; it is a disease that a cardiologist might diagnose once in their career.

Brian and I went to Jonathan's office, and he talked to both of us about what it meant to have ARVC. I sat there listening, hearing only part of what he said. Tears were running down my face, even though I was trying to hold them back. I didn't even realize I was crying until Jonathan handed me a box of tissues. Brian asked questions; I did not. No one wants to feel any of the feelings I was having, but feeling them all at once was excruciating. Brian was amazing. He did everything he knew to do to console me, but I still felt lost.

Jonathan went on to tell me that I definitely needed surgery as soon as possible to put in an ICD (implantable cardioverter defibrillator — a small device that's implanted in the chest or abdomen to treat arrhythmia). That is when I felt the anger finally stirring inside me. I didn't want an ICD. I felt like I was losing control of my life. I told him no. He tried to explain that both he and Zoubin were on the same page about this and that I needed one. I stopped listening.

The entire drive home, I cried in silence as I stared out the window of our car. It didn't feel real. A few months ago, that felt like a lifetime ago, I had had no worries. I was the mother of an amazing one-year-old, working in a job I loved, and training for my first half Ironman.

That night, I wrote in my journal, "I am scared. I am

confused. I am sad. I am angry. I feel lost. I feel powerless." I was feeling a lot of emotion and wasn't sure what to do. I couldn't run away from it. I now knew for sure that was no longer an option and never would be again. Running and triathlon had made me who I was, but they had also contributed to me developing the heart disease with which I had just been diagnosed.

I'm not sure if it was the same day or the next day that I spoke with Zoubin. He confirmed that I needed to get the ICD immediately. I told him I wasn't getting it right away, that I couldn't. I pushed back against both my cardiologists because I needed time to process what was going on.

Against their strong recommendations, I waited a little longer. I didn't wait until I was ready because, honestly, I might never have been ready. Instead, I waited until I could simply bear the idea, if not accept it. A week later, I booked a trip to Mexico with my best friend, Nora. I remember the look on both Zoubin's and Jonathan's faces when I told them. They weren't happy, but I think they understood.

So a few weeks after starting my own physical therapy practice, and a few weeks before planning to have ICD surgery, I went to Mexico, and I am so glad I did! Mexico was a blessing. I was able to stop and assess what I was going through. I was able to process. Nora and I spent hours and hours talking, laughing, and crying. We had an amazing time. We took a yoga class while listening to the ocean, we read books on the beach, we fell asleep in the hammock, and we walked and talked and reconnected. It was exactly what I needed. When I got back, I scheduled my surgery.

At the same time all this was happening, we had our son

tested. The day we went to get the test performed was a difficult day for me. It was the day I realized the gravity of the situation. Prior to our appointment, I hadn't really processed what was happening. We found out that Andy had a 50 percent chance of having the PKP2 gene — in other words, a 50 percent chance of developing the same disease I had. A 50 percent chance of never knowing what it was like to run, bike, or swim. A 50 percent chance of sudden cardiac death.

That was also the day I realized that my disease was, in fact, progressive. I had heard it a million times, but it hadn't sunk in until the genetic counselor said it out loud again. All I could think about was how I wanted to be here for Andy, how I wanted to see him grow up, how I wanted to grow old. I didn't want to be depressed, angry, or tired all the time. I realized how much I wanted to be present for every moment I got to spend with him. No matter what happened, I was going to make sure I was around for him as long as I could possibly be — hopefully for years and years to come.

The very same day we met with the genetic counselor, I also had another stress test. I failed it. And I cried. It was all too much in one day. I had secretly hoped all the work I was doing to calm myself down and to change my lifestyle would help me improve the condition of my heart. I kept holding on to the idea that this was all a bad dream. Until now, everything that had happened in my life I had been able to fix or change. This was the first time I had ever felt truly powerless.

I don't pray that often, but that night I prayed that my son didn't have the gene. I didn't want him to have to live his life scared that something might happen. I didn't want him to lose the chance at playing on a team and learning the value of sports. I didn't want his life to be restricted in any way. I had always dreamed we would run races together and eventually get him on the kids' triathlon team. I knew none of that could happen if he had the gene.

I also wrote in my journal that night to clear my head. In big, ugly letters I wrote, "This sucks! ARVC sucks! I miss running. I miss the freedom and peace it brings. I miss my pants fitting. I miss having energy. I miss sleeping through the night. I miss drinking red wine and eating chocolate and drinking caffeinated coffee and living without fear. . . Look up yoga studios and call a personal trainer."

7

The End of Running

"This may not be what you wanted, but beauty often grows from discomfort."

- Mandy Roberts, Owner of Form Yoga

Before I left for Mexico, there were several months when Brian and I didn't talk much about what was happening. We tried, but I was still in a place where I couldn't easily communicate how I felt, and neither could he. I know this is why I felt so alone sometimes. I had a difficult time letting anyone in, even him.

Our entire world was being turned upside down. I was no longer able to help at home and with Andy as much as I wanted or we were used to. Many of the things we had always shared together such as running, being active, spending time outdoors, going on adventures, or going out to eat at nice restaurants were much more difficult. I didn't feel like the person he had married. I didn't have the energy, and I was really struggling. I felt more and more alone every day. It felt like we were just trying to survive.

Brian was under a lot of stress at work and tried to let his company know what was going on with us, but it was difficult. When a family member has cancer, everyone understands what that means. When someone has a rare disease like ARVC, people don't know what to say, how to act, or what to do. He thought telling them I was having health issues would create more support and understanding at work, but unfortunately that is not what happened. Rather than being supported, he was made to fear he might lose his job if he asked for too much help or wasn't 100 percent all the time.

During these months, Brian was often late to meetings because he had to drop Andy off or go to an appointment with me. Initially, he tried to explain but didn't feel heard, so eventually he stopped explaining. He was told he was missing the mark left and right, and he felt criticized and misunderstood. No one he worked with had any idea what it was like for him at home, and although many people asked how I was, only a few reached out to ask Brian how he was. Despite caring, there was little effort made to help lighten his workload. If he had been in a place where he knew how to ask for help, he probably would have, but in the middle of chaos, it is difficult to know what you need.

I could see how difficult it was for him because he has a lot of pride in his work and, like many people, his work is a huge part of what defines him. He was there for me, but that meant when Andy and I went to bed, he stayed up all night working. He was burning the candle at both ends. When I had my ICD put in he was working on his computer during my surgery and while I was recovering in the hospital. He was trying so hard to support me but didn't want to lose his job. I think a lot of people who have partners at home who are sick go through something like this. Our society doesn't allow weakness and vulnerability, especially in business. His company is one that prides itself on their support of work-life balance for their employees and putting their people first, but they failed. This put a lot of stress on Brian, our family, and me.

When I got back from Mexico, even though I had agreed to get the ICD, I didn't want it. I fought it. I was angry with my doctors for telling me I needed it. They were right, but it scared me. It meant the ARVC was real. It made the fact that something serious was wrong with me very real, yet again. It meant I had to accept that my life wasn't going to go back to the way it was before. Initially, I got it for Andy. And I got it for Brian. I didn't want it for me.

Once my surgery for the device was planned, I began telling my family that I needed an ICD and that surgery was scheduled. I told my mother first, and she wanted to come down to help. She was so upset that I didn't want her to come. She turned my struggle into a story she told herself about how I didn't want her to be a part of anything in my life. The truth was I didn't have the capacity to take care of myself or anyone else, especially her. If I was going to get through this, if I was going to survive, I couldn't let it be about anyone else.

After many conversations with my mother, I called Shawn,

hysterical. I was distressed about upsetting my mother, and it brought to the forefront so much of my anger around my childhood. I had worked so hard to get away from feeling not good enough and from being responsible for everyone else's feelings, and here I was, momentarily right back where I had started. Shawn guided me to a place of reason and coached me to stand my ground. She reminded me that I had to do what was best for me and my family and not anyone else. I wasn't responsible for how my mother felt. She was.

Then I called my father, but he didn't say much. He never says much, but I wanted to scream at him, "Say something! Anything!" I didn't feel like he cared, even though deep down I knew he did. I was upset he didn't offer to come down and help, but I also didn't tell him I needed him. I don't know why I didn't just say, "Can you come help us?" I wasn't in a place where I felt comfortable enough to ask for help, even though I really needed it.

Then I called Naomi and Holly. They were former patients of mine with whom I had become very close over the several years I had treated them. Even though I was their physical therapist taking care of them, as time went on, it seemed more like they were taking care of me. If I looked tired, suddenly a coffee would appear.

When I got pregnant and still hadn't told anyone, somehow they already knew. And when I finally did tell them about Andy, I think they may have been more excited than I was. On holidays, they always send cards and gifts, even though I never expect them. Whenever a package comes in the mail for Andy that doesn't have a name on it, I can correctly assume it is from them. They call just to say hello and make sure we're doing okay. They've always been there for me to talk to no matter what. To all my friends in Atlanta, I refer to Naomi and Holly as "my moms."

A few months before my surgery, they moved from Atlanta to Bethesda, Maryland. When I called them and let them know what was happening, they didn't ask me if I needed help. They simply told me they were coming, and, before I knew it, they had booked their flights. That was exactly what I needed, and Naomi and Holly knew it. They knew me so well that they knew what I needed without me asking.

However, even though they were there to help us whenever we needed it, as were Brian's parents, I still felt like no one around me understood what a big deal the surgery was to me. Getting the ICD was about more than just surgery. It was the end of my life as I knew it. Even though the internal defibrillator was meant to save my life, that's sure not what it felt like to me at the time.

One night a week before surgery, while I was making dinner, I started to think about my will and how I hadn't itemized all my jewelry and belongings that I wanted people to have. I ran down some of the list in my head. Andy should get my engagement ring, my niece Adeline my favorite diamond and blue topaz earrings, Jenn all my cycling equipment. The list went on and on, so I decided I needed to write it all down before my surgery, and I did.

When I would hear my son laughing, I found myself wondering if I was going to die on the table in surgery. I wanted to hear that laughter again, and I was so frightened I wouldn't. When I look back now, it seems like I was being a bit melodramatic, but at the time it sure didn't feel like it. My fear was very real. I had experienced so much disappointment, and my life was filled with so much uncertainty, that I often assumed it was the worst-case scenario that would actually play out.

I managed to suppress my feelings about the ICD surgery right up until the morning it was due to take place, December 18th. I had been so angry that I never gave myself a moment to let everything sink in. Anger was blocking all my other emotions. I suppose that is the nature of an athlete. As an athlete I had learned how to push through and keep moving toward my goals regardless of the course ahead. I had been just trying get to the finish line, to be over the nightmare.

That morning, as soon as I was taken back into the pre-op area, I started to cry. I tried not to, but I couldn't help it. I just couldn't stop crying. Everyone recognized me, but this time I wasn't in a joking mood, and I could tell they felt sorry for me. Zoubin came in, and as soon as I saw him, I cried even more. My vision was blurry, and tears were streaming down my face. I was trying so hard not to feel, but I could no more stop my feelings than I could stop my tears.

Zoubin sat down on the edge of the hospital bed, handed me a tissue, and said nothing at first. Then he told me he too wished I didn't need to have the surgery, but quickly followed up with, "But you have to." He kept sitting there on the edge of my hospital bed, handing me tissues as my tears kept falling faster and harder. He never rushed me. He just sat with me until I was ready.

The surgery was difficult. I didn't expect it to be so painful. When I woke up, the first thing I did was feel where I knew the device was implanted. Yet again, I was hoping it was all a bad dream, and yet again it wasn't.

My ICD isn't a typical one. I have a subcutaneous ICD that is located in my armpit. The wires don't go into my heart, but around it instead, and they are embedded in the breast tissue. The location isn't very visible from the front, but it sticks out from my armpit a little in the back.

Right after surgery, under my arm and along my side were very swollen and uncomfortable. I couldn't turn over in bed, and it was difficult to get in and out of bed. I had to brace myself and have Brian help me. Breathing, coughing, and laughing all hurt.

I refused to take the pain medication because I didn't think I needed it. I wasn't afraid of the pain. When Zoubin came to check on me, he asked about it, and I told him I didn't want to take it. He laughed and said something like, "You are so stubborn." Of course, he was right. I was being stubborn. I hate medications because the smallest amount typically affects me a great deal.

Even though I was in pain and getting out of bed was so difficult, I still spent the next two days walking the dreary hospital corridors every hour or so unless I was sleeping. Moving felt so great! I wandered up and down the halls in the middle of the night, wondering, "Is this real?" I was the youngest, fittest person there, and that made my whole situation seem so surreal. But I was much calmer and less angry. I was moving into the stage of acceptance.

The car ride home from the hospital was horrible. I could feel every tiny bump in the road and every single turn. I had a difficult time leaning back comfortably in the car seat because it put pressure on the surgical site. I had to sit slightly turned to the right and cross my legs to the right to help take the pressure off. I wanted to cry. Of course, it was partially my fault because I had refused the pain medication at the hospital.

I didn't think that I would want or need help when I got home from the hospital, but I was wrong on both counts. I was so exhausted physically and mentally that I was very thankful when we got home that we did have help, even though I had told everyone I wouldn't need any. Luckily, Naomi and Holly hadn't agreed with me and had come anyway. I was so exhausted and so out of it that I needed to be told what to do, and they were up to the task. They took charge in their loving but no shit kind of way!

After several attempts, Naomi finally convinced me to take a little pain medication because I could barely move without help and was clearly struggling. She was right, of course. Even though it knocked me out, I was able to sleep, and I could move better and tolerate the pain more. Naomi also helped me wash my hair because I couldn't get the bandage wet or lift my arm. It's amazing how much better clean hair can make you feel!

Holly made sure we all got fed, that Brian wasn't losing his mind, and that everything was under control. My in-laws took Andy for a few days so I could rest, and many of my friends and patients brought us food. They were all so amazing. I had always been the one to help others when they needed it — to take care of them whether they liked it or not. I wasn't used to being the one who needed help. I felt so vulnerable and unsure in this new role.

After Naomi and Holly left, I called Jenn to help me wash my hair and shower. There are only a few people I would let help me with this, and she drew the lucky number! At this point, I was starting to feel a little better, so at least we were able to laugh at the situation. I even called my friend Melissa, and she came right over to check my scar and change my bandage for me.

Leading up to the surgery, I had stopped talking to a lot of people and was even unpleasant to some. I didn't do it on purpose, but I was protecting myself. The less I talked about it, the less real it seemed, and the less I had to reassure others that I was fine. Despite this distance I had put between myself and others, so many people took the time to help us.

However, even though we ended up having so much help, the weeks following surgery were more than difficult. I got a serious virus that made me feel even worse. It made me even more tired, and it was even harder for me to get out of bed. I was in a lot of pain, and it was very emotional. Brian was overwhelmed with managing work, Andy, and everything that was happening with me. It didn't help that it was Christmastime.

I love the holidays. Every year I get so excited for Christmas I usually change the pillowcases on the couch to holiday themes, pull out the holiday books, make hot apple cider on the stove, sit by the Christmas tree just to look at the lights, and give tons of dinner parties. But this year I couldn't have cared less about the holiday. I didn't want to see anyone. I was in too much pain, and I was drained.

I was also self-conscious when people came over to visit or drop off food. It was difficult for me to get up off the couch, and I couldn't wear a bra because it hurt too much to have anything touching the scar. It was unseasonably hot for December. So rather than being somewhat hidden and comfortable in bulky sweaters, I was forced to wear revealing tank tops.

The day after Christmas, I woke up very early, sat straight up in bed, and couldn't catch my breath. I started crying for no reason and finally, several minutes later, settled back into bed. Then a few hours later, just as the sun was rising, the phone rang. It was my brother. I knew something was wrong because it was early and his voice was quavering. When he could finally get the words out, he told me that my mother's mother, my nana, had died that morning.

I screamed and began sobbing uncontrollably. Brian ran to my side, but it took several minutes for me to get the words out. It hurt so much in so many ways. The sobbing made my side hurt even more, and emotionally I could barely handle it. I had been very close to my nana. I spoke to her every week. She was the first person I called when something good or bad happened in my life. She had been a rock for me growing up and someone to confide in as I became an adult. I have never cried as much as I did that day I learned of her death. I couldn't stop.

Even though I felt horrible and had been lying on the couch or in bed for several days, and even though I was still emotionally drained from both the surgery and Nana's death, I wanted to go to my grandmother's funeral. I really felt like I had to be there. So I called Zoubin, and he said I could fly since it was nearly two weeks after the surgery. I really wasn't in good enough shape to fly, but we flew home to New York anyway.

Flying was strange because, not only did we have our eighteen-month-old to negotiate in the airport, now I wasn't supposed to go through the metal detector, and I couldn't lift anything at all. Everything from that week is a blur. My physical pain had subsided some, but I was emotionally drained.

I think that if I hadn't gotten sick after surgery and if my nana hadn't died, my memory of getting the ICD wouldn't be so bad. However, December of that year was a month in which nearly everything that could have gone wrong did. But we still made it through. I kept telling myself that it had to get better, that there was nowhere to go but up.

It took longer than we thought it would, but finally, a month later, I was back at work and slowly feeling better. The first week back was a bit challenging because my job is very physical. My arm was still hurting, and wearing a bra was uncomfortable, but I could do it. The more patients I saw and the more time that passed, the better I felt.

It was getting easier because we knew what we were dealing with, and many difficult things were behind us. I finally started to feel like I could move forward in my life. I began enjoying things again and even talking to friends. It wasn't perfect, but it was progress.

Having the ICD was strange. Initially I was bothered more by how the device felt than what it looked like. If you didn't know I had an ICD, you probably couldn't tell, especially in winter when I was wearing heavier clothing. The device felt like a pack of playing cards was in my armpit, and I couldn't let my arm rest against my side. I noticed little things like it was uncomfortable to put anything under my left arm, bras didn't feel good when they touched the ICD, and sleeping on my left side remained uncomfortable for several months.

I never thought my scars would bother me, but they did. I have a large scar under my arm that is several inches long and another one under my left breast, near the sternum. I found myself staring at them in the mirror and trying to decide how I felt about them. Some days I didn't mind, and other days I would suddenly start crying and cover up quickly with a shirt.

I was really bothered by how my device and scars looked when I put on my bathing suit for the first time. I didn't want to go to the beach. The scar was visible because it was large, and the ICD stuck out quite a bit. I was more self-conscious than I'd thought I would be. Now I am not as bothered by it as I was in the beginning. It took me a long time to realize that most people don't even notice it.

I didn't anticipate the wardrobe changes that would come with the device. I had to give up wearing some of my favorite dresses that zipped up the side because they no longer fit with my ICD. I got rid of a lot of the clothing that didn't work anymore, but occasionally I still find an item I thought I could wear but can't.

For many months, I tried wearing the same sports bras or regular bras I used to wear. However, eventually I realized they didn't fit as well anymore because the ICD was big enough to increase the circumference of my chest. It annoyed me because I was already self-conscious about my body. If someone didn't know better, they would think the ICD was fat sticking out of my bra. When I finally decided I had to get new bras, it was nearly eight months later! I waited too long and put myself through so much unnecessary discomfort. Not only did the new bras look better, they felt so much better.

One February day, a couple of months after my surgery, I tried to run. I had been told I could try it, as long as I ran slowly for just two to three miles a couple of times a week. I thought, "Great! Now that I have this ICD, I am safe." I was wrong.

I went out slowly and ran at a twelve- to thirteen-minute-per-mile pace, walking all the hills. Most of the anger I had felt a few months earlier was gone, and I was so happy just to be out there putting one foot in front of the other. I thought to myself, "Okay I can do this. It doesn't matter anymore how fast or how far I go, only that I can."

As I ran, I smiled from ear to ear. I thought about all of the people who go through terrible things and, once they are on the other side, find their way back to running. I was elated and positively giddy.

My plan was to run one mile and then walk, but it felt so good I just kept running. The air was cool, and the sun was warm. The sidewalk was a little wet from a passing storm, and drops of water continually dipped off the trees and landed on me. I was jogging down a long hill, taking my time and listening to everything around me. I could hear the birds singing and the cars passing. The smell in the air was crisp and damp. I was feeling great, and I stopped at the bottom of a hill to walk up it.

My Garmin started beeping, and I looked down at my watch. My heart rate had jumped up from 125 to 198 BPM. I hadn't felt any palpitations, shortness of breath, or other strange feelings, so I was surprised. It really scared me. My ICD was set to activate at 200 BMP, I sat down on a curb, put my head between my knees, and tried to breathe. I wanted my heart rate to come down. I didn't want to get shocked!

I cried. I was terrified of getting shocked, and I was frustrated because, once again, my heart wasn't doing what I wanted it to do. I hated that feeling of having no control. There was nothing I could do.

Eventually my heart rate came down, and I didn't get shocked. As I watched the numbers go from 198 to 160, 150, and finally down to 90 BPM, relief washed over me. I sat on the side of the road for a long time, tears streaming down my face. I had made so much progress. I was rarely angry anymore. I had been taking time for myself, and I had stopped pushing my body and myself so hard. I felt betrayed by my body once again. Finally, I stood up and walked slowly home, defeated.

I never tried to run again. There were a few times I thought I would try. However, every time I thought about it, I got so scared and anxious that I would get palpitations. The idea of going out there with the possibility of being shocked was worse than not going at all.

Then, later, when I finally was getting up the courage to get back out there, I learned that even running a little bit can possibly cause faster progression of my heart disease. The research demonstrates a correlation between disease progression and how much people with ARVC continue to exercise. The more exercise, the faster the progression. The choice to stop running became less about what I wanted to do and more about being here for my family in the long run.

It has been very difficult for me to let go of something that has shaped and defined me for so long. I still have vivid dreams about running and competing in triathlons. I often wake up in the morning and remember each step I ran in my dream. I can hear the crowd cheering. I can feel the wind on my face. I can taste the sweat. Then I realize it was only a dream.

I hope that running will come back to me someday but, if not, I recognize what it has done for me. It has been the catalyst for who I have become, and for that I am eternally grateful. I have come to realize that perhaps I've learned the lessons I was meant to learn from running, and now I am meant to learn new lessons.

I've always been competitive. Losing my outlet for my competitive nature has been incredibly difficult. When Shawn brought up yoga as an alternative to running, I wasn't convinced. When I lived in Boston, I used to do Bikram hot yoga twice a week at five in the morning. I loved it because it always cleared my head, and I felt like it was making me a stronger runner. As a runner, I always thought of yoga as a way to stretch after a long run. It was a supplement to my "real exercise," which was running, cycling, and swimming.

To satisfy Shawn, I did online yoga classes at home, watching an instructor. I always felt good when it was over, but I found myself trying to get through it as fast as possible, and I was distracted and unsatisfied. It was clear that something was missing, so I gave it up for a while. I told myself yoga wasn't for me. Since I had never considered yoga real exercise, it's probably true that I wasn't giving it a fair chance.

Then one day I finally decided to go to an actual yoga class at a local studio with my friend Julia. She had been trying to get me to go with her for a while, but I always had an excuse. However, I eventually decided that I had to do something. Yoga was something I was allowed to do, so I'd better give it another shot.

I walked into the studio thinking, "I'm not sure about this. Do I really belong here?" I only knew one person in the class and wasn't comfortable with yoga. Then the music came on. It was gangster rap, and I began to laugh. All of a sudden, all my preconceived notions of what yoga was supposed to be were shattered, and I fell in love with it immediately. The class was too hard for me, but I did my best. More importantly, it was fun and made me laugh. I was hooked.

I started going once or twice a week, and then a few weeks later they announced they were having a forty-five-day yoga challenge. The goal was to complete thirty classes in forty-five days. I thought, "Perfect! I can do this!" My husband jokes that I found the only yoga studio in Atlanta that has competitions.

At first, I too thought of it as a competition. I calculated how many classes I could do and plotted how I could beat everyone else. As I began to take more classes and meet more people in the yoga community, I realized it wasn't a competition at all. It was motivating me and forcing me to further explore myself physically and spiritually.

I now go to yoga anywhere from three to six times a week, depending on what my week looks like. It hasn't replaced running, but it is helping me redefine who I am now. I have found another amazing community of which I can be a part. My studio, Form Yoga, is like a family. After I was there long enough, I got to know people and hear their stories. There are so many amazing people that surround me with so many incredible stories, I only have to ask or listen. If I hadn't stopped running, I never would have become part of this community, and I would have missed out.

The other day in class, we were all in a posture that had many levels of difficulty. Of course, I wanted to do the best I could, so I was uncomfortable in the pose and pushing hard. Then my teacher Elizabeth said, "I invite you to reevaluate your foundation. If you ease up, you may find that it is easier to breathe."

It clicked. What she said allowed me the space to back off and feel good in the pose. And it made me realize that I had been doing the same thing in my life for so many years. Pushing as hard as I could in my career, in my running, in every aspect of my life. No wonder I hit a breaking point. No wonder my body broke down. I wasn't listening at all.

8

All in the Family

"Let the fear teach you instead of paralyze you."

- Dr. Shawn Haywood

It's no secret that I didn't enjoy being pregnant. You lose control of your emotions, your body, and sometimes even your mind. To say I complained a lot is an understatement. I think the hormones made me evil.

However, despite the fact that I didn't like it, I did everything I knew how to do to positively impact my son's growth in utero. I talked to my belly, and I listened to classical music as much as I could. Brian and I read books to my belly at night, and I exercised every day, running up until I was thirty-six-weeks pregnant. Everything I did, I did to make my son, Andy, smarter, stronger, and healthier.

I didn't take any drugs during labor because I didn't want anything to affect his little body, and perhaps just to prove to myself I could do it. I breast fed for nearly fifteen months, despite the fact that it was painful, and I hated pumping. I did it because the research I had read indicated that babies who are breast fed have higher IQs. Most mothers are determined to give their children everything — love, a good education, the benefit of their hard-won wisdom. I was no exception. I certainly never planned to give my child disease or heartache.

Right when I felt like I was finally getting my feet underneath me again after my diagnosis, my son tested positive for the PKP2 gene. This is one of the many genes that have been discovered to be linked to ARVC*. I had known that Andy had a 50 percent chance of testing positive, but I had convinced myself that our family had gone through enough. That he would be just fine.

When Erin, our genetic counselor from Children's Hospital, called, I was the one who answered the phone. I was in the process of driving to a coffee shop to do some work and was almost there. I certainly wasn't ready for what she had to say. In my mind, there was no way Andy had the gene. It simply wasn't a possibility.

The moment she uttered the words "I'm sorry..." I couldn't breathe. I couldn't speak and tears started rolling down my face. I had to pull the car over. I heard her ask me if she could do anything, and I was unable to answer her. Instead, I sobbed and sobbed and finally hung up the phone.

I was paralyzed. I sat in the parking lot across from the coffee shop for a long time, not sure what to do next. Finally, I called Erin back. She suggested we bring him in to the Children's Sibley Heart Center for baseline testing.

When I thought I had finally collected myself sufficiently, I called my husband. But the moment Brian answered his phone, once again I couldn't breathe or speak. Every word I managed to make come out of my mouth was uttered as I sobbed and screamed. I was inconsolable and incomprehensible. But even though Brian couldn't understand a word I was saying, he instantly understood what was going on. He told me to meet him at home, that he would leave work immediately.

I could barely see as I drove home, and I felt like I was being strangled. When I walked in the door, I fell onto the coach and curled up in a ball until Brian arrived. When he got there, he just sat quietly with me on the couch as I cried, rubbing my back and running his fingers through my hair.

It took hours for me to stop crying. I'm crying right now as I write this, and I've had to get up from the computer three times before I could keep writing. Knowing that I gave my son the gene for ARVC has nearly killed me, and every time I think about it, I get nauseous. I feel responsible for ruining his life before it even got going. Hearing your son has the one thing you never wanted him to have is crushing. It's as if all the breath has been sucked out of your chest, and you are suffocating. All the emotions, pain, and grief I experienced about my own diagnosis were nothing compared to this news and my reaction to it.

The next day, I made an appointment at the Sibley Heart Center at Children's Hospital in Atlanta. The first time we went, we had no idea what to expect. Both Brian and I were anxious, and I couldn't sleep the night before. The office is much like any other doctor's office, but it is lighter, happier, and has a lot to distract the kids.

Everyone at the Sibley Heart Center was wonderful. They were so kind and answered all our questions the best they could. They told us Andy was the youngest child they had ever encountered in whom they had discovered the gene, and there was no protocol for what to do in this type of situation. They decided to do a baseline EKG and clinical exam, counsel us on what they did know, and then plan to bring him back yearly for observation since children his age almost never show signs of ARVC. When they put the EKG stickers on my son's little body, I could feel the tears welling up in my eyes. Brian held my hand and entertained Andy, making a game out of the test and exam.

Since that first visit, we have been back just once, and it was a little easier. Shawn helped me realize that Andy doesn't understand the seriousness of the situation. Going to the cardiologist is normal for him, so there is no reason to make a big deal out of it. Now when we go to the doctor's, Andy expects to get the stickers on his chest for the EKG, and he likes to check out the stethoscope. At home, he has a white doctor's coat and kit and pretends to be a "heart doctor." He makes us call him Dr. Edwards and who knows? Maybe someday he will be a heart doctor for real. He doesn't have signs of the disease now and hopefully never will.

When we brought Andy home after he was born, he was wrapped in a receiving blanket that said, "Born to run, 26.2, half marathon, keep running..." I used to dream about doing all the kiddy races with him and eventually running with him at 5Ks, 10Ks and the triathlons for kids. This will never happen.

According to what we currently know, if Andy were to become a runner, his chances of getting the disease would be

80 percent higher than if he chose a life without endurance sports. The reality is that we won't do races and go to these events like I had planned. In fact, we won't be cheering for him at any sporting events. There will be no running, cycling, swimming, soccer, basketball, or any competitive sports. I come from a family of athletes. It never occurred to me that my child wouldn't have the chance to be one. His life will be filled with other things instead. Amazing things, but not what I had imagined. Maybe he will be a musician or an artist or play golf.

Before he could speak, Andy was already noticing all the athletes surrounding him, and every time he pointed out a runner or a cyclist I would cringe. Andy is three years old now, and when he spots any of our friends running down the street, he cheers them on or yells to them. He loves to watch races — bike races, road races, and triathlon events. At Ironman Texas, we couldn't pull him away from the transition station. He kept yelling, "Look at the bikes, Mom!" When he sees sneakers, he asks me if they are my running shoes. He always wants to "run fast" and race down the street. It is so difficult to hear the love of running in his voice when I know I can't let him pursue that passion in the future. Recently he has been racing his friends. He has perfect running form, and the smile on his face is pure joy.

I've been told he can "be a kid" right now, but whenever he runs, I get a sick feeling in my stomach because I know I will have to take that joy away someday. I know this will be one of our struggles as he gets older. I recently got a text message from a mother on our street about signing up all the boys in the neighborhood for soccer. I didn't respond. I wanted to, but I couldn't bring myself to explain why Andy wouldn't be participating. It was just too much.

I hope our son understands why we are going to have to make certain decisions around athletics. At Johns Hopkins, we were told to let him live a normal life until about age ten and then to consider steering him away from competitive sports. I am afraid he will hate us for holding him back from things he and his friends will want to do.

I know it will be difficult because, even though I don't run anymore, all our friends run and do triathlon. At our house, we watch the Tour de France rather than football. On weekends we go to races, and my entire career is about endurance athletes. Andy is going to grow up around competitive sports and endurance athletes. At some point, he may choose not to listen to what we have to say. If he is anything like me when it comes to stubbornness and determination, then we will be in for a struggle, and he will challenge us. I can only hope he makes the right decision for his heart, even if that decision means not following his heart.

Once I knew Andy had the gene and I had started to come to terms with what was going on, I wanted to learn as much as I could about ARVC. I was more accepting of what was happening, but sometimes anger would creep in. Some days I would be okay, and then the very next day I would wake up angrier than I had been before. The emotions I kept swinging between were anger, grief at the loss, and acceptance. I felt alone and scared and like no one knew what I was going through. The less I talked about it or acknowledged it, the less it felt like it was happening to me. But I knew that wasn't working. I couldn't stay angry or in denial and continue to move forward with my life.

A few months after my diagnosis, my husband and I went to the yearly ARVC seminar held at Johns Hopkins in Baltimore, Maryland. On our way to the conference, I found out my grandfather had just died, less than six months after his wife, my nana, had died. I was already anxious about going to the conference and having my first appointment at Hopkins, but losing Papa made the week even more challenging and emotional.

The conference is held every year in April. April is a funny time of year because the weather can be warm and beautiful or cold and depressing. It also happens to be when the Boston Marathon takes place. So instead of going to Boston, we now go to Baltimore. The first year we went to the ARVC seminar, it was rainy, cold, gray, and depressing.

Brian, Andy, and I flew to DC so that Andy could stay with our friends Naomi and Holly while we were at the conference. They picked us up at the airport and let us borrow their car. They were very supportive but didn't ask too many questions because they were fully aware of how fragile I was feeling. On Friday morning, Brian and I drove about an hour from their home to my first appointment at Hopkins.

The closer we got to Hopkins, the more anxious I got. I just kept looking out the window and not speaking because I didn't have anything to say. I was hoping they would read all my records and tell me that my doctors had been wrong, that I didn't have the disease. I didn't want one more person telling me what I couldn't do. I had already lost so much control over what my life was going to look like. I didn't know if I could handle another doctor telling me yet again what I had to give up.

As we pulled into the Hopkins parking garage, I could feel the rage and anger building in my chest. "I don't want to be here!" is the declaration that kept playing in my head. I was shivering from the cold rain drizzling down around us and felt as gray and overcast as the sky above us. I had a sick feeling in my gut before we even walked in the door. No matter how many doctors I go to, I still have trouble every time I meet a new one. I still feel the anger and rage build up inside me. I'm not exactly sure why, but I think it's a defense mechanism I use to avoid getting hurt any more than I already have been.

The closer we got to the office, the worse I felt, and the more annoyed I became with everything around me. I didn't like the orange band Security had given me to wear on my wrist. The elevators took too long to come down. Then the check-in was automatic. I had to scan the barcode from my paperwork in the kiosk, and it was supposed to bring up my information.

The kiosk nearly sent me over the edge. "What do you mean I have to check myself in?!" I complained loudly. I was so flustered that I couldn't get the check-in to work the first few times. When Brian tried to help me, I snapped at him. Eventually, with assistance from the administrative staff, I was able to check in. I was annoyed that my appointment didn't start exactly on time. No matter what happened, I was going to be annoyed.

The waiting room was fairly empty, so my tantrum went unnoticed by everyone except Brian. The area was small but had red, green, brown, and blue pleather seats scattered around the room. It was quiet except for the sound of the occasional patient checking in or the printer running in the background, printing out labels for each patient's chart.

Brian and I sat down in two of the blue pleather chairs in the waiting room. I tried to read, but it was hopeless. I kept reading the same line over and over. I felt anxious, scared, and nervous. I didn't know what to expect. I didn't like that Brian was talking to the nurse and she was talking to him instead of me. His jokes made me angry, even though I knew he was only trying to help.

I was just plain angry. About everything. I was angry I was there. I was angry I had this disease. It wasn't fair! Why did I have to have ARVC? I was uncomfortable even just saying out loud that I had ARVC. If I said it out loud, then it was no longer a nightmare. It was real. I didn't want anyone else to tell me I had this disease. I was afraid. I was afraid they would tell me I was much worse than I thought.

That morning we met with Brittany, the genetic counselor, and Dr. Calkins. I was completely shut down, and I know I was rude at first. I was trying so hard not to cry and to just make it through the appointments. I didn't want to be rude or angry, but I didn't have access to any other emotions. I hadn't learned how to deal with my emotions yet.

The ARVC team at Hopkins was fantastic. Despite my anger, despite my blatantly rude behavior, they were caring, empathetic, and knowledgeable. As the appointment went on, I warmed up a little and was even able to smile.

Brittany was great. She had so much information at her

fingertips and was compassionate about everything that was going on. Brian and I asked a lot of questions about the disease, the gene, what the future might look like, and even pregnancy. She was able to talk through everything we asked about without hesitation. She gave us research articles to look at and laid out what living with ARVC might look like. It was not what I wanted my life to look like, but she at least gave us an idea of what to expect.

They confirmed that I did, in fact, have ARVC, but, luckily, I had only mild changes in my heart tissue and moderate electrical issues. Both Brittany and Dr. Calkins said this with a smile, as if it were a good thing to have mild-moderate ARVC. Of course, I knew it was because obviously the less severe the ARVC the better. They were being empathetic and kind and encouraging, but I wasn't ready to hear it. All I heard was "moderate disease," which created a story in my mind that equated moderate with terrible. I just wanted to get out of there.

Then we talked about exercise. I distinctly remember Dr. Calkins saying, "You have a choice. You can choose to stop exercising, and your disease will likely progress slowly. Or you can continue to do what you have always done and get worse much faster." Once again, I was being presented with the idea that the one thing I loved and had always thought was good for me was making me worse. I heard him, but I was heartbroken, scared, frustrated, and angry all at once.

I thought it would be a no-brainer that my family members would want to be tested once they knew about the PKP2 gene connection to ARVC. I couldn't have been more surprised or frustrated when I realized no one wanted to do it. It has been such a struggle to convince them to get tested! I tried to stress the importance of finding out, but no one seemed to hear the urgency in my voice. I sent three different tests out to my family that simply entailed taking swabs of the insides of their mouths and sending them to a lab. I was incredibly frustrated and frightened when my loved ones chose not to be proactive.

Most people with this disease die before they find out. So why didn't my family want to know and prevent premature death? I asked Brittany for advice, and she offered to write a letter to my family. I sent her letter to everyone, and, so far, two people have decided to be tested. Everyone else has an excuse for why they haven't done it yet.

I'm told this is a common problem among ARVC patients and their families. Many of the families that finally have testing done are often ones who wait until after they have lost one, two, or three members of their family. I am frightened that this will happen in my family. That despite everything I have said or done, it will take something terrible to get them to act. I hope this isn't the case. I wouldn't wish this on anyone else.

We left the Hopkins clinic that day with more information and understanding about the disease, but I was an emotional mess. We decided to go down to the harbor, walk around, and get some lunch. The sky was still overcast, and the wind off the harbor was cold. We found a little pub with a few locals sitting at the bar, and we grabbed a table. I didn't talk much, and Brian wasn't sure what to do. We were both a bit in shock. It was a lot to absorb.

That evening, Brian and I went to the ARVC seminar's meet and greet event at the Marriot near the harbor. I was very nervous about attending. I don't really like big crowds, and I definitely don't like crowds of people I don't know. We were a little late, so when we walked in, people were already seated and talking at various tables or standing around commiserating with each other. Then I noticed that each table had a theme — "I have ARVC," "My loved one has ARVC," and "I used to be an athlete." I made a beeline for the table labeled "I used to be an athlete."

I quickly began talking to the people at my table and discovered we all shared the same story, which went something like this. "I have always been healthy and have been an athlete for a long time. I was training for a (marathon, Ironman, triathlon, etc.), and I noticed I was tired all the time. My runs didn't feel like they used to. One day, my heart started racing, and I couldn't get it to stop. I thought I was going to die."

It was the first time I felt like someone else knew what I was going through. We told our stories and laughed at jokes others wouldn't find funny. We talked about our exhaustion, inability to sleep at night, fear of dying, anxiety, our grief at the loss of running and exercise. This evening was by far the best part of the conference. It gave both me and my husband the feeling that we were not alone in this.

Brian and I met a woman from outside Atlanta at the conference. She was there because her son, an avid basketball player, had just been diagnosed with ARVC. We didn't get a chance to talk a lot with her during the conference, but we exchanged emails and eventually got together after the conference, back in Atlanta. It has been nice to have someone in the same city to talk with and relate to.

The rest of the conference offered a lot of good information, but it was overwhelming. The lectures by various people were helpful because it let us know how hard they were researching and working on ARVC. Since the disease is a rare condition, there isn't much money available to support research. So what they have done so far is pretty amazing. In fact, at one point they thought they had cured the disease. However, it was discovered that the cure ultimately caused cancer, so it was back to the drawing board.

Some of the information didn't speak to me or make me feel better. Some of it made me downright angry (Big surprise, right?). They told a story of a young man who had ARVC and kept getting shocked over and over again by his ICD. I kept wondering, "Is anyone helping him manage his stress or anxiety other than via medication?" They spoke about the medical management of the disease, but not much about the holistic management of the patient.

Endurance athletes are driven, overachievers. We want answers and are willing to put the work in to get results. I would have liked to hear from a sports psychologist rather than the psychologist they had speak. A sports psychologist would have been able to talk about what to do when you lose your entire identity and way of life. It would have been great to hear of holistic ways to manage stress, like meditation, yoga, and talking to someone instead of taking anti-anxiety medication.

I felt like there was so much more that could have been addressed. However, it is a small conference, and every year they take attendees' advice and modify things accordingly. I am looking forward to more about holistic care and less about medical management at future conferences.

Even though the conference was an excellent opportunity for us to meet people and learn more about ARVC, I had a difficult time being around it so much. It was all so new to me, and I'm not sure I was ready for it. It was good for me to meet people who were going through what I was going through, although many of them seemed depressed and didn't really know how to cope with what was going on. We were all in the same boat, but it felt like there was no one to direct us down the river.

Going to the conference allowed Brian to connect with other spouses and hear that what he was going through was not unusual. So much of what had been happening all year was about me. There were only a few people who ever stopped to ask him if he was okay. At the conference, he heard how other spouses had so much support at work and at home. I think Brian left feeling underwhelmed with the support his company had given him. When he heard how other spouses' teams rallied around them and supported them, I think he became disappointed with his colleagues.

His family had been great, but we hadn't shared with them a lot of what was going on. We probably could have made it clearer that we were in trouble, but we didn't have the energy or time to do so. Brian was under so much stress, and I couldn't help him because I was barely able to help myself. I was glad he was finally getting the opportunity to talk about what was on his mind with people who were experiencing the same thing.

When we left the conference, we were worn out. It took us several days to relax and recuperate and several weeks or even months to integrate everything we had learned. When I got home that Sunday, I went to a restorative yoga class. As I lay there on the floor in the shavasana (corpse) pose, tears rolled down my face. Instead of feeling ashamed, as I used to when I cried, I felt relieved. I never used to cry when I needed to. I was so proud of being tough. But what I have realized now is that tears are another way of letting go. That night in yoga class, I let the tears roll down my face as I continued to breathe and be present to what I was feeling. When I left the class, I felt better and ready to move forward again.

Since that first ARVC conference, we have been back. The last time we went was much improved because both Brian and I were in a better place emotionally and physically. The weather was sunny and warm instead of dreary and cold. I had coping mechanisms to deal with how I was feeling. On the drive from Naomi and Holly's to Hopkins for my appointment, I closed my eyes and meditated rather than thinking about all the horrible things that could happen. As I looked out the window, I thought about all the things I had accomplished since the last time I had been there.

When we got to Hopkins, everyone we'd met previously remembered our names, from the doctors and genetic counselors to the other families with ARVC. We met more people struggling with our same issues, people who had been newly diagnosed and were feeling how we had previously felt. This time I wasn't as angry and could actually joke around with the genetic counselors, Crystal and Brittany.

When we saw Dr. Calkins, he asked me how I had been feeling, and when I said good, he seemed a little shocked.

Apparently my PVCs (premature ventricular contractions) were higher than most, but I attributed my feeling good to all the lifestyle changes I had made. We discussed running and exercise, and when he asked me how I felt about them, my reply surprised him. I said, "I miss running. I will always miss competing. In fact, someday when I have lived a full life and am really old I just might put a magnet on my defibrillator and go for a run." The next day at the conference, he told everyone what I had said and, even though he hadn't identified me, many of the people in the room already knew he was talking about me!

During the conference, I met someone who had been shocked by their ICD over forty-seven times, a swimmer who had gone into VT and nearly died in a pool, a family that had three kids with ARVC, two people who had run the Boston Marathon before finding out they had ARVC, and many others whose stories were similar to or worse than mine. I realized, once again, I wasn't alone. My feelings weren't unique or unjustified. I also realized how important the changes I continue to make in my life are.

Brittany and Dr. Calkins both agreed it would be more complicated, but it was possible for me to have another baby, even with ARVC. Andy is now at the age where people start asking if we are going to have another child. And even though I didn't like being pregnant, suddenly faced with the idea that getting pregnant again may or may not be a good idea, I am distraught. The older my son gets, the more I want him to have a brother or sister.

However, if we wanted to have another child, it wouldn't

be easy. I would have to have my ICD turned off during labor, so a cardiologist would have to be present. I would likely feel worse for about three to six months following delivery, and my arrhythmias and cardiac symptoms would get worse. One research article indicated that the heart can return to its pre-pregnancy condition a few months later. The truth is no one really knows. This is what I heard. "The pregnancy will be complicated, and you will feel worse. We don't think you will get too much worse, but we aren't sure. And you may pass on the gene to another child."

So Brian and I decided that it isn't worth it for me to get pregnant. It's just too risky. However, that doesn't mean we don't want to have another baby. We don't know. Actually, it's more like I don't know. Brian would have another child in a heartbeat.

I'm afraid of having two children for several reasons. I know our life would change again, and I would have even less control. I understand that the loss of control is a common fear and common truth everyone faces as they decide what they want their family to look like. However, the bigger issue for me is can I handle it? I have really bad days sometimes when I'm exhausted and Brian has to do everything. If we have two children, his burden will increase exponentially. He insists he wants two, and it will be okay. However, it is a real fear of mine that it may be too much. We are so lucky to have the one.

We are weighing all our options. Surrogacy and adoption are both on the table, and each comes with different considerations and risks. I never would have considered the idea of surrogacy, but one afternoon several months ago, my friend Jenn came over for coffee and brought it up. She told me that she and her husband, Scott, had spoken about it and had agreed that, if Brian and I wanted another baby, she would carry it for me. I never even had to ask. She simply offered. That is love.

Since then, we've gone to see an IVF (in vitro fertilization) specialist in Atlanta and begun the process, but we haven't fully committed to it yet. It's a lot to digest. I was completely overwhelmed at everything that goes into it — the hormones, the process, the attorneys, the cost. I have days when I am all in and think, "Let's do it!" Then the next day, I have a completely different mindset.

It's difficult for me to see my friends having second children. I am happy for them but a little jealous. I know we would have been pregnant right now if it hadn't been for ARVC. I love that new baby smell. My friends are constantly laughing at how I sniff every baby's head. I love snuggling and rocking babies to sleep. I love watching them grow and seeing their personalities emerge. When I see Andy interacting with other kids, I feel guilty because I know what a great brother he would be. I don't know where we will end up. I don't know what path we will choose to go down. For now, I am in the middle of processing what it all means.

---

* Other genes that have been linked with ARVC in order of prevalence: PKP2, DSG2, DSP, DSC2, JUP, RYR2, TMEM43 (http://www.hopkinsmedicine.org/heart_vascular_institute/clinical_services/centers_excellence/arvd/symptoms_diagnosis/genetics.html#associated_genes)

9

Letting Go

"We must let go of the life we have planned, so as to accept the one that is waiting for us."

- Joseph Campbell

After many difficult months, a battery of tests, and a sobering diagnosis, I was finally breathing again and this time more slowly and deliberately. I knew what was wrong with me and had a clear picture of what I had to let go of. Shawn was helping me to face many of the issues I had run away from year after year, and I was beginning to come to terms with my diagnosis and what it meant.

Yoga had become a new outlet and a safe place for me. I was building a new community. I loved working for myself, and my company was a great outlet for all of my bottled-up energy and creativity. Brian and I were finding our footing again. We were learning how to navigate our new life together. I was still having some challenging days and nights, but each day and each night got better with time.

A few months after our first ARVC conference at Johns Hopkins, I received an email from Susan, the mother I had met there who lived outside of Atlanta. Susan, her daughter Ann, and I got together for lunch. It was really nice to have someone to talk to who understood what was happening to me and to our family. They were going through the genetic testing for their family and still trying to figure things out. Ann was in high school and being recruited by several big-name colleges to play basketball. Her brother Joe had been diagnosed with ARVC after he collapsed while playing basketball. Ann hadn't been diagnosed with the disease yet but was beginning to face some of the life challenges that come with the possibility of developing the disease at a later date.

I was all too familiar with how they were all feeling — the fear, the confusion, and the sadness. Ann was applying to colleges to play basketball with the knowledge that she might not be able to play. She was describing some of the same physical sensations I had been having. Periodically, she was light-headed or felt her heart jump in her chest. My heart sank as I listened to her, but I continued to hope she tested negative. I thought how lucky I had been to have more years under my belt before I found out. What would my life have looked like if I had been diagnosed in high school? I never would have run marathons or done triathlon. I might never have gone to PT school and met my husband. So much of who I am and where I am in life is because of endurance sports.

About a month after my lunch with Susan and Ann, Ann came to my clinic and shadowed me for a day. She told me that the day before she had found out that she did indeed have

ARVC. Now she had to decide what to do about school and moving forward and said she might be interested in PT school after she graduated from high school.

I was heartbroken for her. She barely shed any tears, but I knew what she was feeling. She was a high school student and handling this with the kind of grace that often only comes with many more years. In fact, Ann was handling it much better than I had. The only thing I could do was give her a hug and let her know she wasn't alone. I tried to share with her what had helped me when I had found out, and I told her about Shawn, yoga, the dietary changes I had made, and meditation. She listened and took it all in quietly, while I tried to answer any questions I could.

Ann is an incredible young woman, and I imagine she will be a source of inspiration for many people someday. Several months after she came to my clinic, I saw her on the local news with her brother, discussing ARVC. I was so proud of her for how she was handling it and how she was using her story to make people more aware of the disease.

It wasn't long after Ann's story aired on TV that I received an email from Polly, a former patient of mine. She asked me about my heart. She had remembered that I was having issues when I was treating her. At this point, I was more used to talking about what was going on so I didn't mind telling her. Eventually it came out that Polly's partner, Janet, was also having some strange heart issues. I invited them for dinner.

When they came and I had talked to Janet for a while, I was blown away by how similar her story was to mine. From the symptoms she had been having to how she was dealing with them. I quickly realized that everyone handles the diagnosis a little differently, but many people go through many of the same things — difficulty sleeping, dealing with the loss of exercise and identity, anxiety, fatigue, feeling isolated and alone, experiencing depression.

Janet talked about walking ten miles in the rain because she couldn't run. I did that. She talked about the frustration of not knowing what was wrong yet. I had been there. She discussed waking up in the middle of the night in a panic. I can't tell you how many times I have done that. Polly described what it was like to love someone going through so much loss and pain. Brian related.

We listened, and I tried to share our story, how I was moving forward, and my knowledge about the disease. I gave them the name of my cardiologists and told them all about Johns Hopkins. When the evening came to a close, I realized how far in my journey I had already come. I also realized that, even though it is difficult and it sucks at every corner, it is better to be here, living with the disease, than not living at all. I still had many unmet goals and dreams, but I was starting to realize it might be okay. Dreams serve a purpose until they don't.

One of my unmet goals was that I had always wanted to do an Ironman distance triathlon, which consists of a 2.4-mile swim, a 112-mile bike ride, followed by a 26.2-mile run (a full marathon). Ever since I had learned what an Ironman race was, I had wanted to do it. For me, it was never a question of "if" but "when."

So many people think it's a crazy thing to do, but I always felt it was the logical next step after qualifying for Boston and transitioning into the world of triathlon. I had never shied away from difficult things in my life, and the Ironman was just another, more difficult challenge to overcome. The idea of breaking down mental barriers and pushing my body to the limit were exciting to me. If someone said to me, "That's crazy," then that meant it was probably what I needed to be doing next.

My plan had always been to do a half Ironman before a full one, but each time I signed up for the half Ironman, it didn't happen for whatever reason. It never occurred to me that maybe I wasn't meant to do one, even though roadblock after roadblock appeared. First, I was sick. Then, I had a concussion. Then, I got pregnant. And, finally, it was my heart.

Even though I wasn't able to compete, Jenn had already done her first half Ironman and then signed up to do a full Ironman distance triathlon in Texas with her brother. We had always planned on doing our first full Ironman distance race together. In fact, when she signed up, I still thought I had a chance of doing the race. I didn't have the training under my belt, but I knew the race was half training and half mental perseverance. I knew I would be fine mentally. Each week I calculated what I could do to train my body. However, as the repercussions of my diagnosis became clearer and clearer, I realized I wouldn't be able to compete.

I finally stopped rewriting my training plan every week and began to realize that I would no longer be able to fulfill my dream of doing an Ironman. Just as Jenn's training started in earnest, I was told I could no longer run, bike, or swim. As she booked her hotel and planned what each week of training looked like, I planned my ICD surgery.

I watched Jenn train, and I was jealous. There she was training for her Ironman while I was still figuring out how to train for watching from the sidelines. I was sad. And frustrated. But I was also excited for her and proud of her.

The training for an Ironman is no small feat. It takes hours and hours of commitment from you, your family, and everyone around you. You have to get up out of bed while everyone else is still sleeping. You have to train in the rain, the cold, and the heat. You have to talk yourself into one more workout, one less beer and going to bed early, even if everyone around you is doing differently. Training is a commitment and a challenge — one that I still crave.

During Jenn's training, we talked a lot about what she was doing and how it was going. I wanted to be as supportive as possible, but it was difficult for me. Every time she went out the door for a long ride, swim, or run, I wanted to go with her. Before I received my diagnosis, I had complained about every early morning run we ever did together. Either it was too early or too hot or both. Oh, what I would have given to be able to complain once again and do it anyway once again.

I had dreaded the days Jenn and I ran to the pool, swam, then ran back home before getting ready for work. Now I found myself craving the feeling of water between my fingers and the smell of chlorine. Training together had been our time to vent, to dream, to laugh, and to be silly. I no longer knew where I belonged. Doing yoga was helping, but I missed my routine and my time together with Jenn.

Now, when I saw my bike, I would sigh or grit my teeth. When I walked by my running shoes at the front door, the tears would come without warning. One day, when I came across my goggles and swim cap in my drawer full of training gear, I threw them across the room.

Even though I knew it would be difficult for me, I wanted to be there for Jenn when she raced. So after many months of training for Jenn and many months of taking small steps forward for me, Brian, Andy, and I went to Ironman Texas. I wanted to be there because it was such a big deal for Jenn. She had been (and continues to be) so supportive of me in so many ways. She had been there to help me no matter what, and I wanted to do the same for her. We were supposed to do our first Ironman together. We were supposed to do *this* Ironman together. I couldn't, but she could, and so I went.

The morning of the race, I got up early and went with Jenn and her family to the start. We were packed in a small car with other people and drove there in silence. Everyone was excited, exhausted, and a bit nervous. It was still pitch-black outside when we pulled up to the athlete check-in, but there were people everywhere. Music was playing, people were laughing and yelling out encouragement, and you could feel the anticipation in the air.

We got out of the car and hugged. I told Jenn I was proud of her and wished her good luck. We stood there for a long time hugging, and both of us started crying. Then I watched as she and her brother walked away, toward check-in. I tried not to be emotional, but I couldn't help myself. I felt like I was being left behind. But that's not what happened.

It had been a very long time since I had been a spectator. I had been so accustomed to being the athlete for so long that it was a very strange and surreal experience to stand on the sidelines, an experience I had long since forgotten. I didn't realize how difficult and tiring it is. It takes a lot of planning to see your athlete on the course in multiple places. There is technology to help you track them on the course, but it isn't always accurate. So there's a lot of packing the car up with signs, racing to one place, packing the car up with the signs again, and racing to another spot.

Brian, Andy, and I managed to meet Jenn on several parts of the course. She did fantastically well in the swim, and we were able to spot her as the mass of splashing water, kicking legs, and stroking arms went by us. We missed her in the transition area but caught her as she whizzed past us on the bike later on. It was so hot and humid for her swim and bike ride. I tried to tell myself, "It's too hot. I wouldn't have wanted to be out there anyway." But I did want to be out there. Instead, I wandered around the course from place to place, taking everything in and trying to catch Jenn as often as possible.

As I was walking quickly from one part of the course to another during the marathon part of the event, storm clouds began to gather, and it got darker and darker. I found a spot by the river, near a bridge to wait for Jenn. Across the way, there were people dressed in SPEEDO swimsuits with their bodies painted, other people decked out in costumes, and a DJ playing music for all the athletes as they ran by. It was so much fun reading all the crazy signs people had written. "Keep moving or I'll vote for Trump." "Real triathletes pee in the water." I spent a long time cheering the runners on as they passed me while I waited for Jenn to appear.

Then, all of a sudden, the rain came. It was like a giant wall of water rushing toward me, and I ran under the bridge for cover. The music stopped, and soon there were no more athletes coming through. They had postponed the race for about an hour because the rain was so heavy and the wind was so strong. I told myself, "Who wants to run in this downpour anyway?" The answer was I did.

I wanted so badly to be out there on every part of that course. I wanted to complain about the heat. I wanted to be nervous about getting kicked in the head on the swim. I wanted my shoes to be soaking wet. I wanted to hate eating another performance gel because it made my stomach queasy. I wanted my legs to be burning so much I could barely take a step. Instead, I waited, huddled under a bridge with at least a hundred other supporters, trying not to get drenched until the race started again. Finally, the rain slowed down, and the race began again. But by then we were all wet, and it no longer mattered that it was raining.

Running had always been my strong suit and swimming Jenn's. So when it came to the marathon, I knew she really needed me to be there, cheering her on as she ran past. And I was happy to be there. The first time I saw Jenn run by, she looked great. She still had a lot of energy and plenty of sass left. Then, as the miles went on, I could tell that the race was taking its toll on her both mentally and physically.

Eventually, I jumped into the race with her. I could tell she was having a difficult time putting one foot in front of the other, and I was having a difficult time watching her in pain. We walked together for several miles. At first, we walked in comfortable silence, and then we laughed out loud. There was a lot of complaining, and I bossed her around about her nutrition as I always have. When Jenn didn't think she could take another step, I made her, and she gave me the evil eye. It was a lot like our training had been in years past. If she felt like running, I took a short cut and met her somewhere else on the course. In total, I walked nearly a half marathon with her.

As the rain poured down on us and it got darker and darker, I was no longer thinking about what I wasn't able to do. And then it hit me all at once, and I suddenly realized what was going on. It was as if Jenn was doing this for me. She said her legs hurt, that they were burning and she didn't want to keep going. I knew she was going to keep going, but she had to say it out loud and let that feeling pass. She was going to keep going for herself and for me.

It was around mile 24 of the 26.2-mile race. It was still raining, as it had been for hours, and it was dark, really dark. Many of the spectators had gone home. It was at that moment that I suddenly remembered what it felt like to be in that much pain. The feeling of complete exhaustion, that your body couldn't possibly go farther, but you had to, and your mind forced you through. I never thought I'd miss that, but I did. So much. I struggled to keep it together, but I started to tear up.

Less than a couple of miles later, it was clear we were near the finish line. The hardest part for me was when I heard the announcer at the finish line announcing all the people who were crossing the line. The closer we got, the more I heard "You are now an Ironman." I had always wanted to hear, "Kate Edwards, you are now an Ironman," but the reality that I never would hear it was very difficult for me to accept.

When we were about a half mile from the finish, I stepped off the course, and Jenn kept going. I watched her run up the hill and through the barricades in the dark. I didn't get to hear my name that night, but I heard the next best thing. "Jennifer Larimore, a teacher from Decatur, Georgia, you are now an Ironman."

When Jenn crossed the finish line, we both cried. I believe she was crying because it was finally over and she had made it, and I was crying for the same reason. As we hugged, she said, "I did this for you." She confirmed what I had suspected but didn't really know until that moment. It was both powerful and humbling to have a friend fulfill a dream for me because I couldn't. I didn't have the medal or the aching body, but thanks to Jenn I at least now had a taste of the experience and the accomplishment.

This dream of mine served its purpose. It taught me that not all dreams have to come true the way you initially imagine they will. I believe this Ironman was another chance for me to let go of something, to shed another layer of my former self so I could continue to move forward. It had been a long, incredible, and emotional experience for me. I was so proud and happy for Jenn. I was also full of sadness because I knew I would never be able to cross the finish line of an Ironman, or any other race for that matter.

The night we came home from Ironman Texas, I went to a yoga class, and I let myself cry. I discovered that the energy, thoughts, and emotions that no longer served me were leaving me through my tears. I was able to let go of what I no longer needed to hold on to. Sometime in the middle of the yoga class, my teacher said something that couldn't have come at a better time. "Let go of attachment. Just because you let go, doesn't mean that you no longer love it, only that you are no longer tied to it."

It was very clear that I had a strong attachment to running and endurance sports. They gave me freedom, courage, and confidence throughout the difficult times in my life. Yet, breaking the link between these sports and myself allowed me to love and respect them without being so attached to them that I couldn't move forward with my life. When I realized this, I felt a new sense of relief because it meant I didn't have to let go of all that I have loved and experienced. I could still love endurance sports and running, even if I could no longer do them. I simply had to give myself the space for new experiences and to be open to loving other things in my life.

Just the other morning, I was in a yoga class, and we were opening up our shoulders. I had a visceral response to the pose. I decided rather than push myself into it that I would go into the child's pose. It was one of the first times in a long time I actually listened to my body. I didn't push it. As I lay there, the teacher came up and put her weight into my back, pressing down into my hips. In that moment, I felt so supported.

I began to cry — something that was becoming more common and less uncomfortable for me. I had been afraid to do the child's pose because of my ICD and my history of shoulder dislocation when under stress. Since my surgery, I had become even more afraid of shoulder dislocation because I thought I would break the ICD leads or have to go through another surgery. I didn't realize I had been holding on to this fear for so long. I let myself cry quietly as I continued to breathe and move through the poses.

Since that class, I have indeed dislocated my shoulder again. It is still horrible and painful, but it didn't break my leads or set off my ICD so I would get shocked. And, even though I was miserable, I was relieved that nothing happened to the ICD. I also realized, yet again, that we don't have complete control over what happens to us, but we do have control over how we respond.

10

Shocked

"Don't let fear take the wheel."

- Unknown

One year after I was admitted into the hospital because they thought I had a heart attack, I went through a metal detector because I forgot I had the ICD. Zoubin had mentioned that I might forget it was there, but I never believed him until it happened. I was going to a baseball game with friends and completely forgot I had anything wrong with me. This was beginning to happen more often. I was no longer consumed by what I couldn't do and started to see what I could do.

As I approached the ballpark, I was distracted and walked right through the metal detector. When I heard the loud beeping, I was confused because I didn't know why it was beeping. I immediately tried to empty my pockets, and then I froze. I realized it was my ICD that had set the alarm off.

It felt like all the blood drained from my face and I had suddenly gone pale. I was afraid that walking through the metal detector would cause my ICD to malfunction. I texted Zoubin. He immediately wrote back and said not to worry, that it would be fine. I laughed and thought, "Maybe it's good I'm starting to forget a little." I had suffered such a large loss of self over the past year that it was a huge victory to forget about ARVC even for a moment.

I was practicing yoga regularly, becoming more mindful about what I was doing in my life, taking more time for myself, and feeling fantastic. I believed I was finally learning to live with my heart condition. I noticed the more I practiced yoga, the more relaxed I was. The more I took part in mindful meditation and acted more authentically, the less often I judged myself so critically.

I found myself breathing louder in yoga class than I used to think was appropriate. I felt the burning in my core and my legs that I never noticed when I was focused on how much it sucked not to be running. Yoga isn't easy — it is a combination of mental, physical, and spiritual work. It was challenging me in more ways every time I let go a little. I think yoga has taught me a lot about myself and my body, and I know it has been my primary place of peace and healing.

As life would have it, as soon as I settled in and started to get comfortable with who I was and what I was dealing with, I was thrown off kilter again. Three days after going through the metal detector at the baseball game, I was shocked by my ICD. All the joy I had about forgetting it was there was gone in an instant.

That morning, I woke up flustered. I hadn't slept very well because I had had a difficult time turning my brain off. I dropped my son off at school and was planning on going to an 8:15 yoga class. I hadn't been in four days, and I was looking forward to it. However, I had forgotten it was the first day of summer camp, so I had to fill out forms and check Andy in. I had even forgotten some of the things he needed on the list they had given us. When I finally finished everything and started to leave, Andy started crying. I never like to leave him crying. I felt like a horrible mom, trying to rush through the check-in and leave so that I could make it to class.

I rushed out of the school and into yoga. Everyone was already on their mat and calmly sitting cross-legged. I ran in, threw my mat down, and let out a huge sigh as I sat down. I was only a minute or two late, but I hate being late. I pride myself on being early and prepared. Once I settled in, I noticed that the studio was hotter than it usually was, probably because the weather outside was getting warmer. I almost asked the instructor to turn on the air conditioning, but I didn't want to disrupt the quiet.

The class started, and it was difficult but felt good. I love to feel my muscles shaking and the sweat on my brow. I knew I was being challenged but didn't think I was overdoing it. I was in a side plank on my left arm when suddenly it felt like I had been punched in the chest. I yelled out an explicit word, lost my balance, and ended up landing on the floor a few feet away.

At first, I didn't know what had happened. Class stopped, and everyone was looking at me. It took me a minute, but then I realized I had just been shocked by my ICD. I was embarrassed but in enough pain and disbelief that I quickly forgot about the embarrassment. I had never been shocked before, and I wasn't sure what to do. I lay on my back and told them to keep going because I was okay. Only a few moments passed, but it felt like forever. No one knew what to do, so they listened to me, and class resumed.

I wasn't okay, but I didn't know what I was supposed to do. My chest hurt, and I didn't want to move. My body was aching from the yoga and from being thrown to the floor. Yoga was supposed to be my safe place — it was something I could do. All of a sudden, everything I had been feeling came up. Once again tears rolled down my face. I was crying because I was frustrated. And scared. And because I had just been shocked and hadn't even been running. I was doing exactly what I had been told I could do. I felt all my old anger return. I thought, "This isn't fair. When am I going to get a break? I've been doing everything right and now this. I've already lost so much. Am I now going to lose yoga too?"

I lay there on my back for about fifteen minutes, tears streaming down my face and my eyes closed, before I was able to pick myself up. Rather than walking out, I got into child's pose. I'm not a quitter. I could hear all the movement around me — the breathing and the balancing — but I just lay there crying. Eventually, as the class was nearing the end, I was able to do some of the stretching while still lying on my back.

I thought I had been shocked because of a combination of things — it was too hot, I was too stressed out, I hadn't had enough sleep, and the class was difficult. My heart rate and rhythm are affected by the weather. The hotter it is, the worse

I feel, which makes living in Atlanta difficult. My heart is also affected by how much I sleep and how anxious and stressed out I am. That's why I had been making so many conscious decisions around how much I worked, changing my lifestyle to decrease the stress and what I took on. And it had worked. Things had been going so well.

After class, my instructor, Jen, came over and gave me a hug. I said I was fine, but my face was red, and my eyes were puffy. Then, without warning, I started to cry again. I told Jen I was frustrated because, "I thought yoga was something I could do." She looked right at me and said, "It is, but we may need to modify it more and turn the air on next time." She was right. She helped reframe what had happened so I didn't leave thinking I could never do yoga again. Sometimes a little perspective is all we need. I am lucky to be surrounded by people like Jen who constantly remind me that not everything is black-and-white.

Before I drove home, I sat in my car with the air conditioner blasting. I debated if I should call someone, and eventually I did. I called Brian first. He was out of town on business in Chicago. Nearly every time something like this happens, he is out of town. Perhaps my body is stressed he is gone, and I don't even realize it. Nothing ever seems to happen when he is home. He asked if he needed to come home, and I told him no, I would call Jenn and Scott if I needed anything. I honestly thought I would be okay in an hour or so. Then I texted Zoubin again. It was the second time I had had to contact him while he was away. He too seems to be gone every time something happens. He at least made me laugh and joked that maybe he needed to consult me before he went on vacation next time.

I went home for a little while and lay on the floor with our dog Austin. After an hour or so of doggy tummy rubs, ear scratches, and snuggling on the floor, I got up and went to my Reiki session I had scheduled a few weeks earlier. Reiki is therapeutic energy healing, and it was one of the things I had started doing about a month after my ICD surgery to help support my emotional and physical well-being. I have found it to be an incredibly useful and supportive addition to my healing toolbox.

My session was with Darshana, one of the many talented healers at The Center for Love and Light, where I work. I knew my time with her would be helpful and that going to my office would be a good choice since my colleagues are so supportive. It was a safe place for me to let go and relax. When we started the session, I couldn't even verbalize any intentions. Darshana understood and did what she thought best. When I left, I felt better, more grounded, and less distracted by what had happened in yoga class.

That afternoon I was exhausted and remained so for several days. My whole body was tired, and my chest hurt a little. However, I suppose 80 joules of power blasted into your chest wall will do that. I kept trying to be "okay" with everything and to continue on with my day as I usually would, but I couldn't.

I tried talking myself into going back to yoga the next day. I even signed up for class online. I was afraid to resume yoga, but I told myself that if I didn't go back right now, I never would. It was rather extreme thinking, but ten years ago I probably would have listened to that extreme thinking and talked myself into going to class the next day, whether I was ready to or not. However, I had clearly grown a lot over the last few years because a few hours later, I realized I wouldn't be ready physically or emotionally, so I canceled my yoga reservation.

I tried to relax and sleep. I was so tired I could barely keep my eyes open but so anxious I couldn't fall asleep. I could hardly get myself off the couch, and all I wanted to eat was ice cream. I felt guilty eating a half pint of ice cream, but I told myself I deserved to eat whatever my body was craving. My guilt slowly dissipated. I watched a movie, and then it was almost time to pick up Andy from school. I began to cry again. I was so exhausted, and I wasn't sure if I would have the energy to take care of him.

I finally called Jenn and Scott and asked for help, something I still wasn't accustomed to doing. I asked them if they would mind picking Andy up. They jumped into action without a single question or hesitation. Scott picked Andy up, and Jenn came to take care of me. I was in a very low place, and they helped pull me out of it. Jenn stayed with me until Brian got home that night, which was a huge comfort. She helped put Andy to bed and then sat with me on the couch as I cried. I am so lucky to have friends whom I truly love and consider family, friends who would do anything to help.

The next several days I was tired. I canceled some patients and saw my doctors. Zoubin was still out of town, so Jonathan went out of his way to get me into the ICD Lab at Emory. When the data from my device was examined, they determined that I had been "inappropriately shocked." In other words, my heart had been fine, and the device had gone off anyway. At first, I was relieved — relieved to know that my heart wasn't getting worse and that yoga didn't cause my heart to go into VT. Then I became nervous and confused. What was wrong with my device?

As usual, Zoubin was great. Even though he was in Europe, he got on the phone with the representative from the device manufacturer and me. They decided that the device shocked me because it was picking up "noise" it interpreted as ventricular fibrillation. They tried adjusting the parameters on the ICD, but none of the adjustments was changing the data. I was then sent for an X-ray to see if the wire in my chest was broken. Luckily it wasn't, but they still didn't know what was going on. They told me no yoga and to make a follow-up appointment with another electrophysiologist so this could be figured out right away.

At my next appointment, they had me doing yoga on the floor of the office as well as demonstrating some of my manual physical therapy techniques, and they were able to reproduce the "noise." They then tried to make more changes in the parameters of the device but finally told me that the entire device needed to be taken out and replaced. In other words, I needed another surgery.

After a week of chaos, I decided I wasn't going to let this send me over the edge any longer. My tolerance for chaos and stress had dramatically decreased over the last several months. The more I made time for myself and took care of myself, the less tolerance I had for getting angry, overextending myself, and feeling overwhelmed. So I allowed myself to be authentic. To be upset, to cry, to rest, to sleep, to grieve until I was done. A week isn't a long time, but that week felt very long. It was enough time for me to pull myself out of the darkness I had fallen into and come back to reality and live.

I went to another restorative yoga class on Sunday night, even though I was afraid I would do something to get shocked again. I was careful and made sure my arm wasn't in a position that might cause the "noise." I am so glad I went! In restorative yoga, we don't push ourselves. Instead, we relax, meditate, and just be. It was exactly what I needed. During class, our instructor, Hannah, said two powerful things, "You have the power to choose your experience," and "Don't let fear take the wheel."

Both of these statements were powerful for me because I realized that yes, I had gotten shocked, and yes, I had to have surgery again, but I got to choose how I would handle it. I could choose to be miserable, or I could choose to be authentic and allow myself to let go. I have a tendency to want to always be in control, but I had been learning that I'm not always going to be in control of what happens. What I can be in control of is how I respond to and handle what happens.

I didn't want anyone other than Zoubin to do my surgery, so I waited until he got home from his trip and went to see him in the office. Once again, I did yoga and demonstrated manual PT techniques to recreate the "noise" in the system. Once he saw what I was doing, he told me that the other type of ICD wasn't an option for me at this point because I would likely break it. He also said he believed the "noise" was being caused by the firing of my muscles around the device, that the ICD didn't seem to be broken. He then sent the data back to the device manufacturer, and together they decided not to replace it. I didn't need surgery! I took a deep breath and, for the first time in a week, felt like I could actually breathe.

Zoubin was able to make some adjustments in the software and told me to go back to my life. The situation wasn't perfect because it was a one of a kind situation. There were no similar cases out there that they knew of, so he wasn't sure if the adjustments would be enough to avoid me being inappropriately shocked. I was elated that I didn't have to have surgery, but I was left with a sense of now what.

Fear reared its ugly head again. I was afraid of so many things. I was afraid something would happen to me, and I wouldn't be there for Andy as he grew up. I was afraid that my husband, as loving and supportive as he had been, would get sick of having to constantly deal with my health setbacks. I eventually choose to acknowledge my fears and then let them go. I didn't want them to control me.

I went to yoga and tried to accept the fact I might or might not get inappropriately shocked again. My intentions for class were to be at peace and to let go of the fear because there was no point in waiting for something bad to happen. It was more important to find the joy and gratitude in the situation and move on. These were all important things I had learned from my work with Shawn.

Even though I continued to put into practice what she had been teaching me, I was still all over the place in the first few weeks following my shock in yoga class. I spiraled right out. Some days I would be okay, but, overall, I stopped watching what I ate, I didn't do much yoga, and I stopped doing Pilates and weight training. I wasn't in a great place. I gained five or six pounds quickly and felt bad about myself for doing so.

Then I went on vacation, and it was perfect timing. I needed to push the reset button. When I got back, I made an effort to go back to yoga consistently, meditate, eat better, and sleep. I quickly began to feel better emotionally, but I still felt off physically. I kept wondering, "Is this all in my head?"

I started to notice that my resting heart rate was in the 70-80 BPM range. Back in my training days, it had been 38 BPM. Then, after I had decreased my training, it was in the 50-60 range. So 70-80 BPM was very high for me. I also noticed I was feeling more fluttering in my chest, and there were moments when I was out of breath and tired. I kept thinking it was still anxiety. I told myself I wasn't doing enough to make myself feel better, so I took more time for myself, got more sleep, and meditated more.

One evening, I was home alone with Andy. As I carried him up the stairs, I felt my heart begin to jump all over the place. When I got to the top of the stairs, I was out of breath, my heart was palpitating, and I was dizzy. I was scared. I was afraid I was going to pass out while I was home alone with my son. I knew what I was feeling was not in my head, that it was my heart. I finally emailed my doctors that evening. They both emailed me back and said to come in the next day, so I did.

It turned out I was having a lot of premature ventricular contractions again. Although anxiety might have been contributing to the problem, it wasn't the major cause of my symptoms. My anti-arrhythmic medication, flecainide, was no longer doing its job. Apparently, it is common for ARVC medications to just stop working. When I was at the conference, I had heard about it happening to several people, but it never occurred to me that that might be my issue.

My doctors decided to change my medication to a new anti-arrhythmic with a small amount of beta-blocker in it, sotalol, and they put me on a forty-eight-hour heart monitor to see what my PVC load was. I immediately felt a positive change in the way my heart felt. I wasn't having constant flutters in my chest, shortness of breath, or dizziness. Success!

Not only did my heart symptoms feel better, but I was even able to ride my bike for the prescribed thirty minutes without having to get off because I was going into arrhythmia. However, I was a bit on the spacey side. In fact, a patient of mine said to me, "Are you okay? You are very chill today. You don't seem like yourself." Of course, I had felt out of it, but I didn't know I wasn't chill the rest of the time!

Then I started to have pounding headaches, and my face broke out in a rash. When I went back to Jonathan, he decided to take me off the sotalol and try another medication. This medication roulette went on for a few weeks because something happened with every medication I tried. Too much sotalol gave me a rash, and I had to drink coffee to stay awake. Flecainide was no longer doing anything for my symptoms. Metoprolol (a beta blocker) made me nauseous, and it was impossible for me to get out of bed. Eventually, we landed on sotalol but cutting the pill in half, and that seemed to do the trick without any complications.

In the midst of getting shocked, changing medications, and trying to get back to a place of feeling good, I had my one-year echocardiogram. As soon as I walk into a doctor's office, I tend to tense up, especially when I'm afraid. The day of the echo, I was so upset that I barely spoke. I was so afraid the echo was going to show I was worse. In fact, I was anticipating that that's what the result of the test would be.

As I lay on the table during the exam, I tried not to cry. When I finally did go to speak, I burst into tears. I asked Sandra, the technician, "How bad is it? Am I worse?" She hugged me and said, "No." Once again, I left breathing a little better but still on edge.

Then I saw Jonathan, and he told me my heart function was better one year later than it had been the year before. That's right — better! It wasn't a huge change, but better is better in my book. I wasn't feeling better, but my heart function was better. What I was feeling wasn't the result of getting worse. It was a result of the medications, my thoughts, my emotions, and my level of stress, all of which are very important factors in ARVC. It was empowering to think that, the more I work on these aspects of my life, the better I might feel.

At my next appointment with Zoubin, he asked me if I thought I was going to get worse, and I responded, "Yes, of course I am because this is a progressive disease." He looked at me and said, "Maybe you won't." He pointed out that there isn't enough research out there right now for us to know my prognosis for sure. He went on to explain, "Who's to say you won't get better? We don't know what happens to this phenotype when you take away all the stressors. Who's to say things can't get better and heal?" He pointed out that everyone is different and that what we know now isn't the whole picture.

I suspect he didn't know the impact our conversation that day had on me. It gave me a lot of hope and forced me to again think about how I framed my thoughts and actions. I realized he was right. We don't know anything. ARVC is a disease that hasn't been researched enough to truly know what's going to happen next.

11

Today

"If there is no struggle, there is no progress."

- Frederick Douglass

This journey has been life-changing for my family and me. The last few years have been a whirlwind, and they haven't been easy. We have been through a lot of heartbreak, tears, anger, frustration, and pain. I am not the same person I was a few years ago. I have had to change so much about my lifestyle, my identity, and my dreams in order to move forward.

I have changed the way I work. I have changed my diet. I have changed my thoughts and beliefs. I have changed my lifestyle. Meditation, yoga, and finding balance have been really important for me during the healing process.

The path I took to get here is not one I would choose for anyone, but I dare say I am now living a life closer to the one I've always wanted. I am surprisingly more relaxed (most of the time), work less, and play a little more. My husband and I are closer than we have ever been, and I can find joy and gratitude in things that once drove me crazy. Overall, I do really well with most of the changes I have incorporated into my life. However, I do get knocked off track from time to time, and, when I do, my body feels it.

As a physical therapist, I specialize in the treatment of triathletes and runners. People often ask me how I can keep treating my athlete patients even though I'm not able to participate in any sports. I honestly don't know. I think that I love endurance sports so much that being part of them in any way I can is actually helpful to me. Every facet of my life is related to being an endurance athlete. Endurance sports are in my blood, and they made me who I am today. I can't change that, and most of the time I don't want to. Some days it's more difficult than others. On the difficult days, sometimes I cry. On the easy days, sometimes I laugh.

In my profession, you get a lot of credibility for understanding what it is like to be an athlete. Not only do I understand what it is to be an athlete, but I also understand what it is to lose everything. I've always been an athlete, and my personal identity has been tied to athletics for as long as I can remember. People trust you when they know you identify with them and understand the intricacies of their sport. My patients feel better when they hear I too am a runner and a triathlete. And they eventually ask me why I no longer race. Sometimes I feel like I have to explain why, and sometimes I don't. Sometimes I explain what has happened, and sometimes I just can't.

There are times I feel like an imposter in my own world. I find myself questioning my own competence to continue to treat athletes because I am no longer one. I no longer race. I no longer train. I worry that I am going to miss things or that I will become obsolete because I no longer swim on my lunch break, run after work, or cycle on the weekends. Every year, the technology changes — the watches, the bikes, the trainers, the goggles, and the shoes all improve. I find myself wondering what will happen when I can no longer keep up with the newest, coolest power meter or running watch because I can't use one anymore.

I am adjunct faculty at Emory University and teach a semester-long course called The Endurance Athlete. I developed the course while I was out on maternity leave. I wrote the proposal, and it was accepted at the same time I had just started to notice something was wrong with me.

Every week for sixteen weeks, I talk about how much I love endurance sports and how to help people return to them when they have been injured. I have a series of guest lecturers, including my sports cardiologist, Dr. Jonathan Kim, and a sports psychologist. I added Dr. Kim after I was diagnosed because I wanted more health care practitioners to be able to screen for cardiac disease in athletes. Physical therapists, for example, have the unique opportunity of spending a lot of time with their patients. They are perfectly positioned to recognize when something isn't right.

In my course, Dr. Kim discusses how to identify possible warning signs in patients. The truth is, athletes are often overlooked because they are so healthy. I was overlooked on more than one occasion and was lucky not to die because of it. I have to admit it is a surreal experience to sit in the room and listen while Dr. Kim talks about rare but deadly cardiac diseases in athletes, one of which I have.

Later in the semester, the sports psychologist comes and talks about how to help athletes handle injury, pain, and the loss of their athletic identity. The first time she spoke, I realized being an endurance athlete was my identity. She was talking about me. Then I wondered, "But I've lost that identity. What stage of grief am I in? Denial? Acceptance?"

I love teaching the course, but it can be difficult. I cried when I watched the motivational Ironman video I had on one of my slides. Brian heard me from the other room and came to just sit and be with me. There were no words for what I was feeling. All I could do was cry. I wondered if I should even teach the class. I wasn't sure I would be able to.

I lecture about running at local running stores, private clinics, and nationally. I stand in front of ten, thirty, eighty, or a hundred people and confess my love of the sport I can no longer pursue. Then I teach my audiences either how to become stronger, faster, less injury-prone runners or how to treat injured runners.

I recently did a clinic for people who were going to start training for the Boston Marathon. I was describing the course in detail, every uphill and downhill, every turn. I talked about specific exercises that would help them race the course better. My eyes started to fill with tears as I demonstrated proper running form. I was able to hold my tears back, and I don't think anyone noticed, but it was hard. The hardest part was being able to describe the course so well, knowing exactly how to race it, but also knowing I would never have that opportunity again.

When I was preparing for the clinic, I put together a group of videos for the participants to watch later. I thought nothing of it when I went to record myself demonstrating how to do the exercises. But when I tried to do some of the plyometrics (exercises where muscles exert maximum force in short intervals of time with the goal of increasing power), I was wiped out. I couldn't do them without having my heart rate jump up and getting out of breath. I did one set of box jumps (jumping on top of a box from a standing position on the floor) and had to lie on the floor for about ten minutes until I felt better.

I hadn't realized I wasn't going to be able to do exercises I had done so many times before. I was so pissed off at my body! I felt like it had betrayed me. I couldn't even demonstrate the exercises I wanted to give people. It was one of the first times my heart was limiting me in the execution of my profession. I was so frustrated, angry, and sad all at the same time.

I work in the medical tent of several running races — the Peachtree Road Race, the Atlanta 10 Miler, and the Atlanta Thanksgiving Day Half Marathon. Every year, the same group of people works in the tent, and it is a great experience collaborating with all different medical professions. Working in the medical tent at the Peachtree is always harder than running the race. We see everything from scrapes and bruises to people having to be transferred to the hospital. It's always hot and exhausting for both the medical staff and the runners.

I have been in so many medical tents on both sides of the

cot. I have been the runner hooked up to the EKG machine, waking up, and wondering where I am. I have been the runner who refuses to go to the hospital or thinks they are completely fine when, in fact, they are not. And I have been the healthcare professional trying to convince a runner to please sit down and let us take care of them.

Most of the magazines I get, the paintings I had made for my office, the books piled on my bedside table, the clothes folded in my drawers, have something to do with running or triathlon. I've started to replace the books on my bedside table, but I still haven't cleaned out all my drawers or gotten rid of all my gear. I'm simply not ready to let go of it yet.

Just the other day, I put on a pair of shorts, and there were safety pins attached to the waistband. They still had attached to them the tops of GU packs I had eaten during a long run. I had been too lazy to rip the GU pack tops off and throw them in the trash, and now they were staring at me. I wondered what run I had been on. Was it a long run from my house to the other side of town, or was it a run where I had driven out of the city to meet a friend, or was it a race? I don't know, and I probably will never know. Some things are just too painful to remember.

My friends are all athletes. And even though I love my friends, there are times when I can no longer relate. There is rarely a conversation that doesn't mention training or an upcoming race or a past race. I like to hear their stories, but I miss not having my own stories.

I had a Tour de France party a few days after my cardiac ablation. As I looked around the room, there were five people who had completed full Ironman races, four who had qualified and run Boston, and nearly everyone else ran, swam, or biked in some capacity. This is my world. But it's a world in which I'm no longer an active participant. I no longer run, swim, or bike. I can no longer sweat or get my heart rate up. And I miss that world. I miss it every day. I miss being able to talk about a crappy run or a great race. I miss dragging myself out of bed at five in the morning to run with Jenn. I miss complaining about it being too hot, too cold, or too rainy. I miss all of it.

Running and endurance sports have given me a lot. I am who I am now because of the experiences I have had. The career I chose, to be a physical therapist who specializes in working with athletes, was the right one for me, and it still is. I love what I do. I love my patients and my friends, and I want to cheer for them in races and hear their race stories. Some days I can, but other days I can't.

Adjusting to my diagnosis wasn't easy in the beginning, and some days it still isn't easy. However, every day I wake up, I choose to be happy, to be grateful, and to move forward. There are moments I still get frustrated and overwhelmed. There are times I feel terrible and completely exhausted, but I am learning how to manage every day.

Running was my only coping mechanism, and it was taken from me. I have been forced to discover other ways to navigate life and manage my emotions. Desperation has allowed me to move forward and grow beyond the constraints I had always previously believed were there. I have discovered that the constraints society puts on us and that we put on ourselves aren't real. We can choose what we do next; we can choose who we want to be. I was pushed off the cliff, but you don't have to wait to be pushed. You can gather your courage and make the leap to choose what to do and who to be. I survived the leap and realized it's all going to be okay one way or another. That's true for you too.

Despite my new outlook on life, just like everyone else, sometimes I still grapple with my identity, sleeping through the night, fear, anxiety, stress, and loss. I have never been a graceful person. In fact, I got a concussion in ballet class when I was young! However, I have tried to make the transition from endurance athlete to yogi as gracefully as possible. I am not super woman, but I do have super powers. They are perseverance, gratitude, and the strength to keep moving forward.

I struggle with fear and anxiety. They seem to be what I struggle with the most, and they creep in when I am vulnerable and let my guard down. Sometimes I am fearful of dying and missing out on my son's life. Sometimes I am fearful of getting shocked again when doing yoga or practicing PT. When I feel a flutter in my chest or see my heart rate increase on my Garmin, I am anxious that something bad is going to happen. My doctors tell me that I will probably be here for a long time and that I shouldn't worry about being shocked or dying, but I do worry sometimes because I am human.

I know that, if I am more present, the voice in my head can't take over as much. I am working on this, but I know it will be a while before I have mastered it. I understand why I can't let fear stand in my way. Emotionally, I can recognize and walk away from my fear about 75 percent of the time, but the other 25 percent of the time I can't.

I struggle with loss. Yesterday I had a Reiki session with Darshana. I went in thinking my intention for the session was to experience peace within and clarity. But before I knew it, I was talking about running again. I was explaining to Darshana my continued desire to put my running shoes on and run out the door. As I sat there talking, I got emotional all over again about losing running. She said, "It sounds like you are describing a dear friend." I was.

At the Hopkins conference, we were told that it is important not to dwell on what you can't do and focus on what you can do. This statement made me so furious when I first heard it. I was sitting in the lecture hall, and I could feel my fists clench and my face flush. I didn't want to recognize I was going to have limitations. Now I can swallow it a little easier and even say it to others.

In fact, that day at the Hopkins conference, they included in a presentation a list of all the approved categories of exercise. Their intent was to help us figure out what else was out there, but telling a serious athlete that they can no longer play basketball, mountain climb, run, bike, or swim, but they can participate in archery and riflery is almost insulting. There is nothing wrong with either of those sports, but a room full of endurance junkies don't want to hear about them. Over time, I have begun to figure out what I can and can't do. I am sure my list will continue to change and morph over time as I relearn my body and as research about ARVC expands.

I have discovered an entirely new idea of what life can be rather than what it should be. I wish I hadn't been so stubborn and had learned these lessons without losing running in the process, but I don't think that was ever an option for me. My body kept telling me something was wrong, and I kept ignoring it. It took me nearly dying before I was able to actually listen to my body.

Although I do what I can safely do given the restrictions of my disease — meditation, yoga, Pilates, weight lifting, bike riding, walking — I continue to love running. I know that the current research doesn't support running for people with ARVC. But I still have hope. I still have hope that someday I will be able to run again, even if it is only a mile or two. What I said to Dr. Calkins at Hopkins is still true. Maybe when I am an old lady, and have lived a full life, I will put a magnet on my ICD, lace up my running shoes one last time, and run out the door.

But today I have a lot of love, hope, and gratitude. Every day I wake up is another day I get to put my feet on the floor and move forward.

About the Author

D r. Kate Mihevc Edwards PT, DPT, OCS is a physical therapist. She lives most of the year in Atlanta, Georgia with the loves of her life, her husband, Brian, son, Andrew, and their Weimaraner, Austin. Since her diagnosis of ARVC, she has had to give up her life as an endurance athlete. She has used her position as a physical therapist, clinic owner, professor, show host, and now author, to educate other endurance athletes about cardiac disease in the healthy population.

Kate is the owner of Precision Performance and Physical Therapy (PPPT), a concierge-style sports and orthopedic clinic. Because of her struggle to find balance following her diagnosis, she created a work environment for herself and her employees that allows for collaboration, compassion, and excellence without the burnout and exhaustion that often plagues healthcare providers. PPPT's culture of its therapists taking care of themselves first and foremost allows them to better serve their clients. The clinic serves the running and triathlon community as well as anyone with orthopedic injuries. However, it is also known for treating patients who aren't able to get better in other environments. Kate and her colleagues are focused on evidence-based and holistic treatment and strive to improve the profession of physical therapy as a whole.

Kate is adjunct faculty at the Emory University School of Medicine, where she teaches an elective course, The Endurance Athlete, to third-year physical therapy students. Additionally, she participates in research studies involving sports and orthopedic topics. She is currently involved in a research project looking at how typical physical therapy interventions affect running form. She has also spoken nationally about running during pregnancy and postpartum.

Kate recently became the host of *The Whole You*, on The Lighter Side Network. In her show, she highlights how to incorporate healthy practices into your daily life at home, at work, and at play to improve your overall health and wellness. She hopes to help people who struggle with injury, acute, chronic disease, or even everyday life, to find ways to be healthy and happy despite their personal challenges.

Gifts to the Johns Hopkins Right Ventricular Dysplasia/ Cardiomyopathy Program can be made through the Heart and Vascular Institute's website at:
www.hopkinsmedicine.org/heart_vascular_institute/ about_us/charitable_giving/index.html

Or, if you would like to get involved, contact the author at www.katemihevcedwards.com

Made in the USA
San Bernardino, CA
21 May 2018